D1084874

ESCAPING YOUR LOW ENERGY TRAP

ESCAPING
YOUR LOW ENERGY TRAP

Uncommon Solutions
Your Doctor Never Told You About

ANNA MANAYAN

NEW YORK

ESCAPING YOUR LOW ENERGY TRAP
Uncommon Solutions Your Doctor Never Told You About

Published in New York, New York, by Morgan James Publishing. Morgan James and The Entrepreneurial Publisher are trademarks of Morgan James, LLC.
www.MorganJamesPublishing.com

The Morgan James Speakers Group can bring authors to your live event. For more information or to book an event visit The Morgan James Speakers Group at www.TheMorganJamesSpeakersGroup.com.

You understand that the information contained in this book is an opinion and it should be used for educational purposes only and is not intended to diagnose your symptoms or personal health condition.

You are responsible for your own behavior and actions, and none of this book is to be considered legal, professional or personal advice regarding your personal health issues. This book is not meant to be a substitute for individual medical advice or for the treatment of any specific medical condition or disorder. Always seek prompt medical care for any specific health issues and diagnosis for any conditions. What you do for your condition is strictly between you and your health care provider/team.

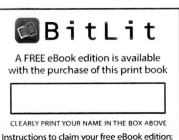

A FREE eBook edition is available
with the purchase of this print book

CLEARLY PRINT YOUR NAME IN THE BOX ABOVE

Instructions to claim your free eBook edition:
1. Download the BitLit app for Android or iOS
2. Write your name in UPPER CASE in the box
3. Use the BitLit app to submit a photo
4. Download your eBook to any device

ISBN 978-1-63047-038-8 paperback
ISBN 978-1-63047-039-5 eBook
ISBN 978-1-63047-041-8 hardcover
Library of Congress Control Number:
2013955193

Cover Design by:
Chris Treccani
www.3dogdesign.net

Interior Design by:
Bonnie Bushman
bonnie@caboodlegraphics.com

In an effort to support local communities, raise awareness and funds, Morgan James Publishing donates a percentage of all book sales for the life of each book to Habitat for Humanity Peninsula and Greater Williamsburg.

Get involved today, visit
www.MorganJamesBuilds.com

Habitat
for Humanity
Peninsula and
Greater Williamsburg
Building Partner

Do not go where the path may lead, instead,
go where there is no path and leave a trail.
— Ralph Waldo Emerson

Table of Contents

FOREWORD

Somewhere between the standardized approaches of Western Medicine and the far fringe of Alternative Healing has been a significant, almost uninhabited, gulf.

Many realize that our generally accepted health care approach is plagued by multiple problems. Driven by profit, a sometimes-myopic focus on acute care and a massive industrial machine, our "disease-care" system, while providing admirable outcomes in certain areas, has been collapsing under its own weight. We are told that, despite spending more than twice what any other first-world country spends on health care, the U.S lags near the bottom of the list of industrialized countries in terms of outcomes. Meanwhile, "modern" diseases continue to explode, with very few good answers coming from our traditional system. This should all be very troubling!

On the other hand, well-meaning alternative practitioners often struggle to find a focus. Is this "complementary" medicine? If so, what is it complementing? Is it alternative medicine? If it is, does it mean the patient must reject the allopathic alternative out of hand? Is it "integrative medicine?" If so, what is being integrated, and how?

Anna Manayan, to my mind, is a good example of a savvy practitioner who understands the scientific basis of health care as well as the intuitive and non-invasive principles of natural medicine. Her determination and scientific curiosity have taken her beyond the typical prejudices found in health care professionals and into the discovery of some remarkably practical keystones to truly holistic healing.

In *"Escaping Your Low Energy Trap"* Anna starts by examining a pervasive condition familiar to all too many in this era. Often misdiagnosed, under-diagnosed and undoubtedly misunderstood, the epidemic affliction of unnatural fatigue saps the creative potential of countless people. Treatments are often haphazard, sometimes harmful and rarely effective in the long term.

The findings in this remarkable little book are wonderful. Although there may be multiple causes, there are also simple keys to understanding, analyzing and treating this pervasive condition. In fact, you may find that discovering the matrix of issues related to this condition can lead you to resolution of many problems you might not even have known you had!

If you're ready to take an unbiased look at a central medical puzzle, if you're willing to become a detective, if you're looking for practical, leading-edge research and answers, this book will open your eyes and will open the doors to enhanced health and vitality. What you are about to read represents a clear, positive note in a cacophony of confusing misinformation and disappointing outcomes.

This is more than hope. It's science with a heart, and *my* hope is that it will find a large and appreciative audience.

—**Grant Clarke**, Co-owner and founder, Energetix Corporation

PREFACE

I want to congratulate you on getting this book, opening your mind and taking responsibility to persistently seek answers for your own health challenges despite what you already hear and know about your present health. Taking this first step means you have initiative; that you have perseverance. Your tenacity will serve you well in getting your health to the next level of wellness!

This book was written to inspire and empower you to seek answers beyond the conventional limitations of "disease diagnosis" that is the bedrock foundation but also a limitation of allopathic (Western) medicine. Knowing its limits you will find new doors opening to provide a broader view on the dilemma of what plagues our epidemic of low energy.

Outside the disease paradigm, health issues can be spiritually, structurally, emotionally, physiologically/biochemically and psychologically based, with mixes of all three! You need not be limited by any one system of medicine's disease only focus or toolbox of remedies. To do so limits your ability to find all the causes for what is keeping you in your low energy trap. This book brings home the pressing need for all our parts to be equally evaluated outside the restrictions of disease references alone. It is only in this manner that we can optimize our energy and thereby optimize our health.

This information is intended for your general knowledge and is presented to assist you in improving your communication and detective work with health care providers. I also hope that the information presented herein empowers you to find answers where none before had been given. It is my hope that in sharing this information, you gain insight into the multifaceted and complex condition of fatigue and begin to comprehend why identifying all its causes is such a challenge for health care practitioners yet alone patients.

A significant proportion of this nation struggles with low energy. Just take a look at the line at the local coffee house in the morning and mid-afternoon. If the cause for low energy were the result of some disease, could there also be significant non-disease contributing factors, factors when not addressed by the allopathic/disease model system leave the patient in a low energy trap? These patients, despite their "medication", have not regained their energy but remain trapped in a perpetual state of low energy. Is that you or someone you care about?

What about those individuals seeking answers yet find no recourse because of the attitudes and comments of their doctors? Comments such as "well that is as good as you can expect" or "you aren't getting any younger". These comments are more common than you think. I hear them every day from my patients. Most individuals are unaware of other significant factors their health care professional is not telling them for lack of time or education that could release them from their low energy trap. It is my goal that you find those missing gaps in the information provided herein.

What does the average person know about the causes for chronic low energy, the type that limits one's lifestyle and causes divorce, school drop outs, disability and unemployment? Most individuals suffering from low energy want to know what they can do to inch forward to improve their energy. Most suffering low energy want to totally escape their low energy prison. They also want to know the causes for why they got there in the first place.

For most individuals their answers are limited to the allopathic "disease" model. Having found one answer, the allopathic doctor often fails to turn over other causes that when added together could significantly outweigh the disease's contributing factor for keeping their patient stuck in their low energy trap!

How much of our plague of low energy is due to a recognized "disease" and how much falls outside this disease model, yet is still medically significant? *Escaping Your Low Energy Trap* is the first book of its kind that examines this overriding health impediment. The question of low energy hasn't been addressed by other published books to date outside of a disease paradigm. Books on specific medical conditions have been written, but not a book that takes a common symptom and examines its uncommon roots as it impacts one's health irrespective of whether the cause is considered a disease, a nutritional deficiency, a medical condition or some other imbalance of the body that manifests itself as indefinitely and cyclically taxing one's energy reserves. Neither has there been a book that examines exactly where our sources for energy are!

People are hungry for answers that will improve their health and help them to step out of their low energy trap. If you or someone you know keeps hitting the snooze button, cannot do the things they use to do for lack of sufficient energy, suffers from a thyroid condition, chronic inflammatory condition such as arthritis, headache, migraine, insomnia, allergies, asthma, Lyme disease, or has failed to recover from a severe cold or flu, is obese, out of shape, overworked, a baby boomers, elderly, or needs to line up at the coffee shop to keep going, then this book is written for you!

Escaping Your Low Energy Trap is written from the perspective of a clinician speaking to his/her patient, who has been plagued with persistent low energy to the point that lifestyle is impacted. It asks the questions that one's well informed doctor should be asking. It answers them with information that the common every day person can understand and use, systematically checking off all possible sources, uncommon sources, presently overlooked by mainstream medicine. The impact of ignoring these uncommon sources leaves one trapped in the unending cycle of low energy.

This book will dispel myths about low energy. Especially, the presumed myth that the thyroid gland is solely or significantly to blame. It provides insight, answers and new opportunities to unveil the hidden causes for one's low energy.

Escaping Your Low Energy Trap is designed to provide a comprehensive view with check off points to solve one's personal mystery for low energy. It will take you on a journey to understand common myths about energy, aging and when low energy becomes a red flag. It walks you through the signs of low energy that are commonly overlooked in medicine and what they mean. It provides you with consequences for ignoring these signs. It identifies obvious and not so obvious culprits for low energy in common lay person terms. It explains how allopathic medicine is designed to miss these culprits. Finally it spells out what you can and cannot do to unveil the cause(s) for low energy. Thus, it is my hope that you come away fully equipped to discuss newly identified cause(s) with an appropriately enlightened health care practitioner. Short of that, it empowers you by letting you know how much you can do on your own and how to access laboratory tests that will act as guideposts for your recovery.

ACKNOWLEDGMENTS

This book came into being as a result of my clinical practice in integrative medicine, Chinese medicine, Anti-Aging medicine, functional medicine, homeopathic drainage, Neurofeedback, functional brain nutrition, and my metabolic immune pathway research. Time and again patients would ask me why their allopathic doctors never told them about the information that I am now presenting in this book, information that I reveal to my patients. They would ask me if I could give them more information in writing about the complex subject of what is affecting their energy. This book is a long overdue resource for anyone stuck in a low energy trap. It is dedicated to my past, present and future patients, and for all those who are looking for answers.

In my practice, I have sought answers to fundamental questions for the cause for certain disorders. The issue of fatigue was on every patient's mind that walked into our clinics. That being said, and acknowledging that medicine is an art as well as a science, I wish to acknowledge each patient for contributing to the body of clinical knowledge that helped formed the basis for which we now successfully treat issues of fatigue.

I also need to acknowledge those who have been mentors and teachers. Your knowledge provided the ladder for new breakthroughs that would not have become possible but for your passion and willingness to share. Your collective knowledge allows countless individuals to benefit beyond the sphere of your personal influence. Everyone in the alternative medical community contributes a part, as we are all connected. However, specific acknowledgment is due to the American Academy of Anti-Aging Medicine, Apex Energetics, Energetix, Epigenic Research, Metagenics, Dr. Scott Walker of NeuroEmotional Technique, and Seroyal, along with their exceptional staff of instructors, researchers, and clinicians who continue to forge new frontiers.

I wish also to acknowledge the founders and developers of technologies that change the face of holistic medicine giving hope to millions: BioMeridian, BioSet™, NAET, Asyra, Zyto, and I2I. Lastly I honor my medical colleagues who have crossed the veil too soon in my opinion. Your influence, contribution, insight, teaching and inspiration helped to remind me that I am a spiritual being serving others and do so from a heart of love and compassion daily as part of my spiritual walk on this earth.

I also honor and acknowledge my fellow medical colleagues in western and alternative medicine too numerous to name. You are all shining stars whose selfless labor and passionate enthusiasm help patients overcome their illnesses. You make me grateful to share this exciting field, ever developing and improving what we can do for our patients.

Besides my patients, teachers, fellow clinicians, medical vendors, and researchers, I need to acknowledge my staff, those presently tolling at Immune Matrix and those who whose time with us was a journey that led to other roads. Your collective enthusiasm for bio-energetic medicine and your patience and dedication to our chronically ill patients, all have contributed to the healing of our patients. Know that your labor has been and is part of the frontier and mission we have to empower each patient to regain their health through natural means whenever possible. You have been and are a part of every victory we make, one patient at a time.

Special acknowledgment is owed to Dr. John J. White, M.D., Chief Medical Advisor Diagnos-Techs™ Inc., Doctor's Data, and Neuroscience

Inc., as this book would not be possible were it not for the bold vision and technological advancements in laboratory testing you have achieved and make so affordable to our patients.

A final and loving acknowledgment to my family and friends whose loving encouragement, confidence and support and unfailing belief in me fueled those long, lonely, dark hours of research and writing often at their expense of my unavailability as a result. Your understanding and faith in me and my research and vision to help patients through education and empowerment is a part of the success of this book.

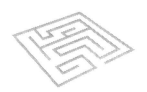

Chapter 1

OUR PERCEPTION
LOW ENERGY

America is experiencing an epidemic of fatigue and low energy. Many blame our busy lifestyles. The sagging economy forces many to work long hours and more than one job. Isolation from our extended families forces us to raise our children alone, isolated from our "family tribe". This puts the sole burden of childcare on the parents, often single parents. But, there is more to this chronic fatigue, this epidemic of low energy our nation is now facing that is not being properly investigated and addressed by mainstream medicine. Why? What can you do to get to the bottom of your fatigue besides chalk it up to aging and lifestyle?

Before we get to the nuts and bolts of this epidemic of low energy and the factors that cause this issue to be perceived as a non-problem (in many cases), you need to have an understanding of the complexities involved in the subject of fatigue as well as its many culprits. Dealing with one cause of fatigue will not necessarily make you whole again. Each piece of the puzzle must be addressed for your body to regain its vitality.

Knowledge is power. Therefore, understanding the medical, social & behavioral factors that impact low energy will empower you to find answers and regain your vitality. Let us proceed to check off all the possible causes for your fatigue so that you can systematically address them and not become a victim of medical oversight!

IS ENERGY JUST A FUNCTION OF PERCEPTION?

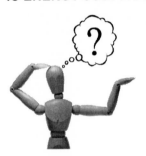

Our perception of health and what that means becomes the bar to which we raise or lower our standards for our personal expectations about health. This is important because perception also influences your health care provider to take action or sweep your "complaint" under the rug. They have their own perceptual bias and it directly affects their incentive and ability to discern your issues as well as provide you with appropriate treatment protocols.

Let's examine how perception becomes a standard upon which to base our personal view of health and guidepost for evaluating health options. Our perceptions become our personal standard upon which we evaluate our cache of energy, and whether we "should" have more. Ultimately, our perception about energy will determine what we do about our low energy trap.

What Is Your Perception Of Low Energy?

Do you accept your current level of energy as "normal" considering your age or lifestyle? Is your perception of "normal" molded by an assumption about declining energy with age? Do you feel low energy is simply a fact of life in the modern world when we all seem too busy to get enough sleep? If everyone you know is tired and doesn't seem to have the energy they'd like, does that mean having low energy should be or is in fact normal?

You and your doctor's perceptions about energy and vitality will dictate you and your doctor's expectations about what you can reap in the area of personal energy and vitality! If you or your doctor believe that as you age you should have less energy, or are victims of modern day hectic lifestyles stemming from long commutes, long work hours, family and financial stressors, then you or your doctor might not look any further for answers. Maybe you have a few health challenges and they tax your energy. Do you feel there is nothing more you can do to improve your energy? Has your doctor told you that?

Knowing your personal perceptions about energy is crucial. Even more crucial is to match up with a health care provider that shares your values and perceptions about energy, especially if you want them to go the extra mile for you to help you regain yours!

WHY IS LOW ENERGY NOT INVESTIGATED AND TREATED MORE?

If social and behavioral perceptions of the public and their health care providers were not enough of a stumbling block to taking action when one suffers low energy, consider this. The public is given little medical education about what low energy means. The public is not educated about when one should seek medical attention for it and when it's indicative of an underlying disease. The public is given no information on what can be done to improve low energy without having to wait to succumb to a disease. Short of a disease diagnosis, patients are not educated, empower or treated "just to have more energy".

Even when a disease is diagnosed, there is little guarantee a patient will be educated about how their disease impacts their energy. Less information is available to empower the patient on what they can do to specifically improve their energy outside the confines of disease management. Bottom line, should we have to wait for a disease diagnosis to be able to do something to improve our energy? Absolutely not! If it's problematic to be advised how you can optimize your low energy while your doctor treats and/or manages your disease, imagine how much harder it is to optimize your low energy when your doctor says you have no disease and therefore tells you that you are "fine".

I hope your philosophy about health is not to wait for a disease diagnosis before you take action to improve your fatigue. I also hope you are not complacent in thinking you and/or your health care provider have done all that can be done to improve your energy.

To understand why there is little support, education, empowerment and thoroughness of investigation regarding the causes for low energy, you need to understand its multiple origins. You must become your own detective, especially on the subject of an "invisible" gland I will speak of.

It is important to become clear in your mind about the focus of allopathic medicine so that you understand its limits. Allopathic medicine (aka western medicine) is designed for the identification and treatment of disease. All the laboratory tests are designed around disease markers, not markers that try to optimize health. That being said, allopathic medicine historically had little incentive to focus on optimizing health or one's energy. This explains why many a patient is disenchanted to be told you are "fine" by their doctor when they obviously feel lousy. Understanding allopathic medicine's focus and objective in treating disease will help you understand its short sightedness when it comes to optimizing health and vitality. It also explains the reason for the limitation in treatment options to that of the disease's "tool box of treatments". It will also help you to deliberately seek answers and solutions outside the "disease" tool box of fixes as would be appropriate when one has a chronic health condition that falls outside a "disease" diagnosis. Your condition is no less real just because it is not a disease!

Some of you have compromised your search for answers at the risk of prolonging your low energy trap in order to have a working relationship with your doctor! You have been brave enough to go to your doctors to broach the subject of low energy only to be told… "It's normal" or "you're getting older now". Some of you have had to endure their suggestions that maybe you are depressed and need a purple pill. If your doctor placates you, makes you feel like everyone feels like that so stop complaining, or that you are fine because they can't find a disease, then how can you possibly hope to escape from your low energy trap?

It may be ok with your doctor to take a pill for every bodily function. A pill to go to sleep, a pill to be able to grin and smile through your day, another pill so your heart beats regularly and a pill so your blood pressure doesn't go sky high, a pill to have sex, a pill to be able to digest your food without stomach pain, or another pill when you get stomach pain after eating anyway, and finally a pill so you can poop, a pill so you don't urinate in bed at night and a pill to keep your arteries open so you don't have a heart attack and can start your day all over again.

In the winter of 2012, I attended a geriatric lecture in Hyannis MA, where it was announced that the average American age 65 was taking four prescription medications daily! Many individuals are on more! In one study, seventy-one percent of the 157 polled reported taking five or more prescription medications. Women took more thyroid replacement, non-steroidal drugs, anti-depressants and anti-inflammatory drugs. Those 85 years or older were more likely to be on drugs for cardiovascular agents, anticoagulants, vasodilating agents, diuretics, and potassium supplements. (Ann Pharmacother. 1996 Jun;30(6):589-95) The Kaiser Family Foundation reported that in 1999 the average retail prescription was 10.1 per capita and by 2009 it had risen to 12.6 per capita. Medical News Today reported in 2011 that 4.02 billion prescriptions were written in American. That boils down to thirteen drug prescriptions for every man, woman and child in American, 13 per capita per day! Do we even eat 13 vegetables and fruits per day? No, but we manage to swallow our 13 prescription pills per day!

What is worse is that our prescription drug "habit" is rising not falling! Our longevity and standard of health is falling. Are we not surprised? That's a sad fact. In 2000, the World Health Organization was the first to analyze and compare health care systems in the world. Of the one hundred ninety one countries examined, the United States ranked 38th in 2000 and has not significantly increased in the 12 years! (World Health Report 2000) Instead the United States continues to slide further down the list.

Bear in mind also that no prescription drug in the United States has been tested by the FDA as safe to be used in combination with another drug or over the counter medication. Yet nearly every prescription drug is at one time or another being used in combination with other over the counter medications and other prescription drugs. Few people know this as they casually mix their prescription medication with another prescribed medication or over the counter medication.

When the FDA approves a drug for public distribution, it means it has only tested that drug's effect alone and not in conjunction with the use of other drugs. In addition, owing to the number of drug recalls and class action lawsuits for "bad drugs", the FDA's rubber stamp on a drug's distribution is NO true guarantee of safety. There is currently no recourse against the FDA for their error in allowing the distribution of unsafe medications! Add that fact to the combined unknown side effects and nutrient depletion of these drugs when used together, and you have a Russian Roulette for deaths, side effects and chronic nutritional deficiencies. All this contributes in some fashion to keeping Americans in their low energy trap.

When allopathic medicine fails to help you find the reason for your symptoms and imbalances, and simply causes you to become pill dependent, then the message medicine is sending you is that it's ok as long as you take a pill to "manage" those symptoms. If that is considered living and healthy living at that, and the underlying cause for why someone needs a pill for every bodily function doesn't raise not one but both eyebrows, then you've got to look where our health care system is going and whether you want to buy into seeing such a doctor for that condition. He or she is simply making you a pill robot.

There is a clear and decisive reason for why the body gets out of balance and develops any symptom. Before you can effectively find solutions, you must become aware of your mindset and that of your doctor's mindset if you are to have any hope of taking the correct road that will lead you to answers. Are you and your doctor of the mindset to be pill dependent "live with it" people? Do you believe that there is a cause, possibly more than one cause, if found could help reverse this downward spiral you are on?

What is your perception of low energy?

Back to perception, let's start first with YOUR perception of low energy. Understanding your perception of low energy and making sure your doctor's view is in sync with your view about energy can make all the difference between you being told you are just getting old (when you are only in your 20's, 30's or 40's) to finding someone that can optimize your energy even when you don't have any disease! Finding a practitioner that shares your view about energy is crucial to begin with.

You have every right to expect and believe that you can improve your energy irrespective of how long you have suffered low energy or a disease, unless you are terminally ill and on the way to hospice. So long as you are breathing your body seeks to heal and regain health, repair and optimize its function. It's up to you to believe in the healing abilities of your body and work towards that goal with health care professionals that also know this truth and are engaged in actively helping people like you to get out of their low energy trap.

Chapter 2

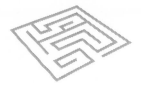

LOW ENERGY MYTHS

L et's dispel the myths caused by faulty perception. Let's dispel the myths that low energy is an inevitable fact of life as we age, or that there is little that we can do to improve our energy even if we do have a medical condition that impacts our vitality and energy reserves.

MYTH 1 – ENERGY IS NOT AN ISSUE AS LONG AS I CAN COMPENSATE FOR IT.

Would you say as long as you can compensate for your low energy and still function and enjoy your life, your low energy is a non-issue? Many of us think we are "fine" as long as we are able to compensate for our fatigue. What many people don't realize is the entire process of compensating for low energy can be a slow slide into a very dark abyss!

I'll give you an example. A medical student studying hours on end to pass exams with little free time, high stress and low energy after having had what she and her doctor/teachers thought was a flu went about her demanding student life coping to boost her energy by drinking coffee. The difference was now she needed to drink double or triple the amount of coffee in the morning just to get going. It became a pot of coffee and it wasn't working so well! She then "had" to drink caffeinated soda mid-afternoon and early evening to stay mentally sharp and study. Soon she needed to add a double shot of espresso mid-afternoon when previously coffee would pick her up alone.

Over time the coffee became less effective and soon it stopped working altogether! She tried to exercise more to boost her energy and stamina but found she couldn't recover as before. In fact, exercise exhausted her now! Her doctor/teachers at the medical school didn't give it much heed. Her standardized blood panels all looked normal and it was chalked up to stress and being in medical school. In fact she was told it is common for medical students to feel lousy during school. It was part of "the test" she was told of who would survive, that "it's the price you have to pay" and that once you graduate you can "get your health back"! So much for teaching our future doctors what it means to be healthy!

Her energy continued to dip into what became the exhaustion phase. Now she felt exhausted after meals. Doctor after doctor said she was fine. One suggested she was depressed! Does this sound familiar to any of you? Fast forward. She had to become her own detective. What she found was not one but three chronic fatigue viruses that had weakened her glands, including this "invisible gland" I will speak of later. Slowly she crawled herself out of the dark abyss and learned a lot in the process. That medical student was me!

We all slip into compensating behaviors until one day
we realize how far we have mal-adapted to our fatigue.

Lay person or doctor, we all slip into compensating behaviors until one day we realize how far we've mal-adapted to our fatigue. Unfortunately, we generally sit up and take notice of our fatigue only when our compensatory lifestyle fails to give us the energy we expect our body should have to get through the challenges and lifestyle of our day.

We compensate by having coffee to start our day. We compensate by having a coffee or soda at lunch, or a double-shot espresso or latte mid-afternoon to counter the after lunch lag in our energy. We eat something sweet when we get tired at our desk at work. All the while we do not realize that if we didn't have coffee, espresso or sweets we'd totally crash and hit a wall and not be able to function.

MYTH 2 – WE CAN AVOID THE DOWNWARD SPIRAL IN ENERGY BY COMPENSATING

Many of us think we are fine as long as we are able to compensate for our fatigue. I thought so myself as a medical student. No one told me how acidic coffee made me. No one discussed diet, or anything **but** disease! In fact the unspoken presumption in medical school was you were fine if you didn't have some disease. Therefore I, like every other person out there, made excuses or found justifications. I had a rigorous schedule and so I thought I was fine as long as I downed my pot of coffee a day just to keep my wheels spinning.

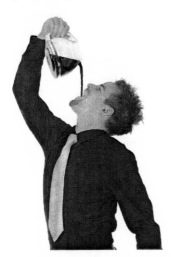

We might compensate for low energy upon awaking by having coffee to start our day. For some of us, a cup is enough. Others need two. Some need that espresso, double, or triple shot! In time, we up the intensity of that compensation by having a latte double shot when a cup of coffee use to work. The espresso in that latte gives us a stronger charge than the coffee use to at breakfast.

For some of us, we find we are still tired, maybe more tired, even with our latte, single or double shot. We add sugar to our breakfast hoping it gives us quick energy. We down a donut, scone, "granola" bar. Any refined carb will do for that hoped for quick energy blast!

As the day goes on, we want to keep our energy up. We find we *need* to have a coffee or caffeinated soda with our lunch. After lunch from 2 o'clock to 4 o'clock we feel a lull in our energy. Off we go to get a double-shot espresso or latte mid-afternoon to counter the after lunch lag in our energy. Some of us get something sweet when we get tired at our desk at work. We hope it helps us have enough energy to finish our day!

Somehow, as much as we might get that pick up, it never seems to last as long as we'd like. Sometimes we crash and feel worse later. This all sounds pretty normal doesn't it? Doesn't it seem most people sitting at their desk feel this way at work? If you don't feel this way I bet you can point to someone around you who does!

As the work day comes to a close we feel too sluggish, drained and fatigued to hit the gym on the way home. Many of us dread the family chores, "dealing" with those high energy kids, and that spouse! It's all too taxing. We just want to relax on the couch a bit (all night if we only could!). Is that normal?

As the evening draws to a close, the kids are in bed. It's you and your spouse now. You feel too tired to interact. You feel drained but you can't sleep. You're sort of wired but zoned out. You haven't had sex in who knows how long because it's all too taxing and who has the time or energy right? Isn't this low energy just a part of modern living and working and raising a family?

If you confide in your friends they will say, "awe, join the club, you're just getting old" or "hey, it's part of working 70 hr. weeks and long commutes". Some more concerned friends might say "Well, maybe you need to get yourself to a gym and get in shape, or go on a diet?" Everyone has an excuse that leads back to the resolution "live with it". But do you have to? Is it truly normal to feel this way?

As life moves onward in our fast pace and we cope with daily living, we ignore these low energy signals our body sends us. More importantly, we ignore our coping mechanisms thinking them a normal part of our daily routine. One day they stop working so well. What we use to do doesn't work to help us get through the day. One day, our coping mechanisms crash and burn. We remain unaware that if we didn't have coffee, espresso or sweets, we'd totally crash and hit a wall. We would not be able to function during the day. It might take some individuals longer than others, but our coping skills will eventually crash and burn and we are forced to look at ourselves with new eyes and hopefully seek new answers.

We only pay attention to the signal of fatigue our body is giving us when our compensatory lifestyle fails to give us the energy we expect our body to have to get through the challenges of our day.

Everything I described above sounds like the typical modern day life and nearly everyone suffers low energy at some time. Nearly everyone compensates for low energy somehow too. What you need to know is why you have low energy because in and of itself, when it occurs daily, and in a pattern that alters your lifestyle (such that you just *have to* have that coffee to function in the morning), then something "not normal" is going on. Something is causing your low energy condition.

It doesn't necessarily mean you have a disease like chronic fatigue or worse, cancer. It is possible, but unlikely. It does mean something is at play affecting the optimum biological functions of your body. It's up to you to become the investigator. Work with a medical "investigator" trained to eliminate *all the causes* for low energy. Don't work with a doctor that placates you into thinking your low energy is just a part of getting old, or due simply to your busy lifestyle, or even worse, suggests off the cuff you must simply be depressed and so you must need an anti-depressant! This book was written to help you check off the culprits and empower you to get real about these symptoms and to get real help.

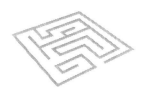

Chapter 3
RED FLAGS FOR
LOW ENERGY

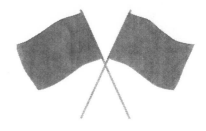

Let's look at the telltale signs. I suggest as you begin to identify with some of these fatigue scenarios, you make a note on paper how many types of situations and scenarios of fatigue you experience, the times of day you have them, and under what circumstances. Then, on a separate sheet list all your coping mechanisms. Unless you know what is going on and how your world is impacted, you won't know how much you could be feeling better!

What are the true warning signs that low energy is something more than being overworked and under rested? When is low energy something we should look into? When is it a byproduct of our lifestyle that we can quickly and easily rebound from with a few adjustments? Finally, when is it the byproduct of sub-optimal metabolic factors (hormonal, nutritional, toxic, and infectious) that have not yet reached a state of "disease" as recognized by allopathic medicine?

Do you wake up tired? Do you wish you could have a mid-day nap? Do you wish you had enough energy to exercise regularly yet alone vigorously? Do you wish you had more energy to play with the kids? Has your energy not been the same since you overcame a recent cold or flu? Do you catch colds and flu more often if you push yourself now? Do you crave sweets for fast energy? Do you find your mind fatigues faster and this then makes your body tired? Do you find recovery from exertion takes longer or it takes less exertion now than in the past to totally wipe you out? Do you notice yourself sighing more or frequently, or encounter times when you feel you can't seem to get enough air despite being able to take a long deep breath? Do you find when you can sleep in, you wake up tired? Does no amount of extended rest or sleep help you feel rejuvenated? If you answered yes to any of the above questions, you are officially in a low energy trap!

Moreover, have you down regulated your lifestyle to compensate for your less than desired energy? Or worse, can you no longer do activities or hold down a full time job because of your low energy? Have you dropped out of school because you cannot study due to your fatigue? Are you unable to cook, clean house, or socialize with friends and family as you once did? If you answered yes to any of these questions, your low energy is *not* normal. You are deep in the low energy trap and can and should act now to reverse the causes that keep you imprisoned. Let's examine in more depth the tell-tale red flags of the low energy trap.

PART 1 – MORNING FATIGUE:

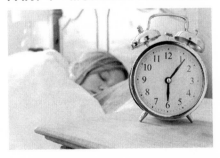

Do you wake up tired regularly? Do you find that when you are able to sleep in you are *still tired*, no matter how long you have slept? Take it for a fact that this is not a normal or healthy sign.

It doesn't mean you have some disease but your body is operating sub-optimally and it can be corrected.

Ignoring your morning fatigue can lead to the progression of a deeper long lasting fatigue. It can lead to the development of more entrenched conditions such as sleep apnea, adrenal exhaustion, syndrome X, obesity, diabetes, allergies, brain chemistry imbalances that lead to anxiety, insomnia and depression, hormonal imbalances that affect your focus, stamina, metabolism, reproductive function and even your sex drive. Ignoring your fatigue can actually lead to disease!

Take a look at the flow chart below to see the connections between low energy symptoms and the development of chronic medical conditions. Also take note for each block in this flow chart there are several prescription and over the counter drugs given to "manage" but not resolve that condition.

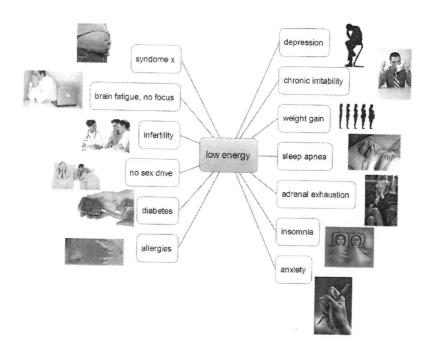

We are not educated by our medical practitioners to realize low energy of the type that requires any sort of chronic alteration in lifestyle or compensatory efforts on our part is a red flag. We are not educated to recognize that such low energy is a big signal the body is attempting to get your attention. It means something is out of balance in your system.

If corrective measures are made at this initial stage, we regain our energy and degenerative, chronic inflammatory processes do not progress. Most importantly, correcting the cause for low energy at this stage is easier than you think! It may take a few months but it's infinitely better than allowing the progressive degeneration of our energy metabolism and fooling ourselves that it's really nothing. The lies we tell ourselves rob us of our vitality and drive that is our birthright, to live a life of optimum health, now and into the future. Don't lie to yourself and don't allow yourself to be overlooked by the medical profession, who are overrun by so called "more important" diseases.

If you are still not convinced regular morning fatigue is something to take heed of and reverse, or you believe you are stuck being this way for the rest of your life read on.

PART 2 – FATIGUE AFTER MEALS:

Some of us suffer fatigue after meals. Meals with bread, rice, potatoes, pasta…carbohydrates make us tired! The more carbohydrates we eat in

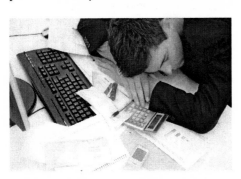

a meal, the more tired we feel an hour or two later. We crave a nap! This is a red flag for insulin resistance and syndrome X.

Test yourself to confirm the level of insulin resistance you have developed. Start by paying attention to how much carbohydrate you eat at each meal. Compare the amount of carbohydrate you had at that meal to the level of your fatigue within an hour to two hours after the meal. On a scale of 0-10, where 0 means you feel great and 10 means you have to lie down to sleep, keep a score of what your energy level is one to two hours after each meal. Also make a note of how much and what type of carbohydrate you ate. For some, any amount of carbohydrate will cause a craving for a nap. For others, a small handful of rice or one slice of bread will cause fatigue!

Test yourself and see. Deliberately eat a meal without carbohydrates. Eat protein and as many vegetables as you want. For example, eat a big tossed salad with broiled wild salmon or chicken. Don't drink any sweetened juices, diet or otherwise with your lunch, and no caffeine, just water. Pay attention to your energy level an hour to two hours after that meal.

Typically, the worse the insulin resistance the more the fatigue after the meal in direct proportion to the amount of carbohydrate you ate. It's best to eat two no carbohydrate meals back to back (like lunch and dinner) and notice how you feel after each meal. Then for the next two meals add your carbohydrates back and compare your energy level.

When you resume your "old diet of carbohydrates" at your meal, notice if that "old" feeling of fatigue returns and how drastic and severe it is. Do you feel sluggish again? Do you need to have coffee? Do you just have to lie down and nap?

If you feel more energetic without carbohydrates in your meal, then it's a sign you have developed some degree of insulin resistance. This insulin resistance is causing the fatigue after meals.

Insulin resistance gets progressively worse over time.

Insulin resistance gets progressively worse over time. One can begin with a slight feeling of fatigue after meals. If and when you eat a big carbohydrate meal, such as pasta dish, you can feel more tired after the meal. Insulin resistance will progress to the point any amount of carbohydrates will cause you to have brain fog, and crave a nap that never rejuvenates you! Due to its progressive nature it's important to deal with it now.

It's also important to take heed other imbalances could be underway. They simultaneously predispose and lead you to develop insulin resistance with ever worsening degrees of fatigue. These imbalances are largely ignored by allopathic medicine. Principally, symptoms suffered by what

I'm calling, our "invisible gland". The optimum function of this gland is largely *ignored* by mainstream medicine. We'll speak more of this later.

PART 3 – MID-AFTERNOON FATIGUE:

Some of us experience a mid-afternoon slump in our energy, anywhere from 2:00-4:00 p.m. We might attribute it to our lack of sleep the night before.

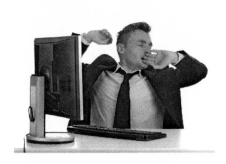

We might blame it on too much work related stress, family stress, late nights or skipping breakfast. We might crave our caffeine boost mid-afternoon to get through the day or reach for our sweet treat for that quick energy boost. We might even crave these carbohydrates and sweets mid-afternoon. Yes, these things can contribute to our experiencing an afternoon slump now and then. However, is this always happening for you? Do you know the actual mechanism, the cause for why you are tired mid-afternoon and regularly? Read on.

PART 4 – WIRED AND TIRED:

Some of us fall into the wired and tired category, especially at night. We are supposed to feel relaxed enough to sink into a restful sleep. Our brain won't shut off, or our body tosses and turns. Again, we attempt to blame it on our work load, worry over kids and family, our job, being out of shape, overweight, or being anxious about life in general. We begin to think this state is normal. Doesn't everyone experience this?

When being wired and tired is chronic, no, it's not normal! It is a sign that if addressed now will prevent the progression of other more chronic degenerative conditions. But no one tells us this.

PART 5 – LACK OF RECOVERY AFTER EXERTION

We all have good days when it feels like our energy is boundless and we go and pack in a full day of activities. However, do you notice that when you've had a full day, the next day you are wiped out? Your energy is so low you can barely make it through a normal day? Are you thinking the grandkids are just wearing you out or you did too many chores around the house? Is it now taking you more than a day to recover from such activity?

Another scenario related to the same *cause* is an apparent lack of recovery from physical exertion. You're out all day shopping, walking all day. The next day you are so dog tired! You might take a bike ride with the kids, something you haven't done in a long while. However, it didn't affect you like it's affecting you now! You just can't seem to bounce back. You are puzzled at the level of activity that induces this fatigue so you hesitate more and more to do the things that you use to do without a second thought.

Sex, don't even talk about sex now because it leaves you drained the next day. You feel heavy, dragging your body through the day. No wonder you enjoy it less and less and it seems more and more an exertion that saps your limited energy reserves.

Your inability to bounce back after normal exertion is a sign that yes, you are in a low energy trap. One or more factors are contributing to keeping you there. In addition, if not addressed, this lack of recovery will spiral downward to limit your ability to engage life as you did before.

PART 6 – DECLINING IMMUNE STAMINA

Along with more frequent bouts of low energy, stamina and fatigue, do you notice that you seem to catch colds easier? Are you fretful when the cold weather comes rolling in that you will catch another cold? Are your colds worse than before? Do they take longer to recover? Did you know that lowered immune vitality is also linked to a common cause...this "invisible gland" that I will speak of later?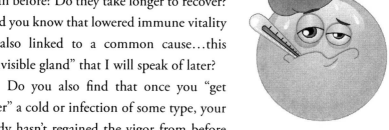

Do you also find that once you "get over" a cold or infection of some type, your body hasn't regained the vigor from before the infection? Do you feel your energy is slowly sliding backwards off a mountain? Do you find it takes more effort and a longer period of time to get rid of any type of infection you seem challenged with. Are you plagued by persistent candida/yeast, sore throats, sinus infections, gut dysbiosis, gum infections as well as colds and flu? These are all significant signs of declining immune stamina that can and does contribute to keeping you in your low energy trap.

PART 7 – MIND POWER WANING

With our drop in energy we may feel an associated drop in mental clarity, focus and stamina. We use to be able to stay on task, think quicker, and longer! Now however, we notice that when our body feels tired, so does our brain. It's as if there is a fog that has rolled in and we don't want to think or do anything that requires focus and attention when our energy is sapped.

All the above scenarios are red flags that should grab your attention that some type of imbalance is at work whose effect can wreak havoc in increasing degrees of severity upon your vitality, your mental focus and acuity, your physical stamina, your libido, as well as your physical recovery and regenerative abilities. These red flags drag down every aspect of your life energy. Potentially, every aspect of your waking and sleeping life can become affected! This is why to ignore the cause(s), is to allow termites to slowly eat away at the very structure of your home, your body.

Chapter 4

EXCUSES THAT LOCK US INTO FATIGUE

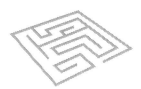

The world encourages us to make excuses until one day we can no longer cope or function. Society tells us to "grin and bear it", "don't complain", "we all have that", as if there was a social taboo about breaking out of our low energy trap! One day we just can't take it anymore. We are forced to see a doctor, someone whose personal views about energy may not be as diligent as you need them to be to uproot all the causes for your low energy symptoms. Do you wait until your car can no longer zip down the road like it used to before investigating why? No way! So why do we wait until our body crashes before we do something?

It's not your fault. Besides cultural taboos have instilled in us our thinking about what we have a right to expect in the way of energy in modern society. The additional unspoken cultural taboo that we should not "question" for fear of appearing to challenge our "all knowing" doctor deters us in seeing our doctor until we truly have to and know we are "sick" or suspect something terrible is wrong. We are discouraged by this

21

medical system to seek their consult when our biological systems seem sub-par when we are told we are fine when in fact we know we are not.

This is no way to educate or empower people to have optimum health by encouraging people to see doctors once their condition is so bad they cannot cope on their own or they suspect they now have some disease or permanent condition! We should not wait until we have a disease to address a symptom, condition or chronic state in the body. We need to be educated and empowered how best to optimize our health and forestall the progression of our symptoms. You, right now, are one of the lucky few who are thinking outside the box, looking for answers!

Could there be more going on? There seems to be little motivation in allopathic medicine to optimize biological function before disease states set in? If allopathic medicine can convince us we are powerless over our symptoms until we have reached a disease state, then allopathic medicine has control over us. We will reach a state of ill health in which we are forced to take whatever fashionable prescription drug is touted for our condition for fear that we will get significantly worse. We will be told that this drug is our only means to control our symptoms. As a result, we will become drug dependent, because the traditional tool box of allopathic medicine is surgery, talk therapy or prescription drugs.

We support the drug industry by ignoring our symptoms until they progress into a semi-permanent state. Is it no wonder why the attitude of allopathic medicine has changed little in the last 75 years? Allowing a condition to progress to a disease requires lifetime prescription drug management. Now that is lucrative!

It pays to let people think they are powerless to do anything about their symptoms, and it pays well!

Can you see the disincentive of Big Pharma to ignore proactive efforts to prevent the development of disease states and conditions that would otherwise require drugs to control their symptoms? Once you have developed a disease, state or condition, fear is instilled to trigger you into thinking your disease has backed you up against the wall and you have no recourse. We all know of someone whose allopathic doctor made these threatening, fear inducing statements in an attempt to goad and manipulate them into submitting to prescription medication as their only recourse:

- if you don't get this vaccine you will get this dreaded condition
- if you don't take this statin drug you will not be able to control your cholesterol
- if you don't take this hypertension pill your blood pressure will not come down
- if you don't take this steroid your arthritis, colitis, any "itis" condition will not be controlled
- if you don't get these allergy shots you will always suffer seasonal allergies
- if you don't take this hypertensive medication (when you don't have hypertension) your heart will get progressively weaker
- if you don't take your aspirin daily you will have a stroke or heart attack
- if you don't take this prescription your osteoporosis will get worse
- if you don't take the seasonal flu shot you will get the flu
- if you don't take this prescription you will never recovery from depression
- if you don't take this steroid prescription drug your eczema, asthma, lupus, arthritis, colitis, etc. will never go away and/or it will get worse
- if you refuse to vaccinate your child for xyz, your child will get it and suffer badly
- if you don't take this seizure medication you will always have migraines, or seizures
- this prescription drug is the only treatment for....

These are some of the untruths allopathic doctors tell their patients to manipulate them into buying into the prescription drug solution. In fairness, some patients have waited too long. Their condition is so severe and/or threatening they need the immediate intervention of a prescription drug. In such cases these drug are wonders. However, in most cases of early signs and developing disease states, prescription drugs do not solve the condition and often mask and enable its progression because the root cause was left to flourish. Worse yet, the prescription medication gives the patient false hope and belief they are being taken care of and their condition will not worsen. Worsen it will if the underlying causal factors are ignored while symptoms are merely managed.

One has to take into account the significant monetary incentive pharmaceutical companies and doctors, yes doctors too, have in turning a blind eye to prevention and early natural intervention. Effective prevention and intervention eliminates the need for all these drugs, especially long term, if only we take action to stop our symptoms from progressing. Can you understand why we are not encouraged by those industries (that use TV commercials whose sole purpose is to sell a prescription drug by telling you what medical condition you should tell your doctor you have) to be symptom free and avoid the necessity of becoming prescription drug dependent? There is no money for Big Pharma to encourage us to be proactive with our health. Rather, they want to brainwash us into telling us what our condition is, giving us the name of our condition on TV so that we can tell our doctors we need their purple pill.

Did you know that sometimes the name of the condition advertised on TV doesn't exist in the diagnostic medical codes? How does the FDA allow this? How is it possible that a pharmaceutical company can fabricate a name for a condition, put it in a TV commercial and tell you to tell your doctor that is what you are suffering from? Furthermore, the TV commercial tells you to go see your doctor and ask for the medication specifically, that little purple pill for example! What is more incredible is many a doctor will oblige you by whipping out their prescription pad after talking to you for two minutes and say just try it and see how you feel. Since when is the medical standard of practice one of experimenting on one's patients? I cannot tell you how many of the patients I've seen go through rounds of prescriptions where their doctors say try this or this or that and wait to hear from the patient if they feel better.

If you think this attitude of reaping profits to sell prescription drugs is only the bastion of Big Pharma, let me share with you what a mother told me. Her son was scheduled to have ear stent surgery (a tube is inserted in the ear to help the ear infection drain) for chronic ear infections. When he came to see me, he had the worst case of ear infections I'd ever seen. He had pus oozing out of both ears! I was shocked and concerned his hearing would be damaged as was his pediatrician, who promptly scheduled ear stent surgery in two weeks.

I asked his mother to give me one month to stop this infection and his cycle of repetitive ear infections. I also asked her to postpone the surgery one month. She agreed and within two weeks, when her son would be having surgery, the infection had already significantly resolved. His mother was delighted and surprised! She returned to her pediatrician for their pre-operative checkup and the doctor demanded to know why she postponed the surgery. When her doctor realized her son's ear infection was now gone, he was shocked and asked why, what had happened that he didn't need surgery. She told him about our clinic and our system of treatment in boosting the immune response to infection naturally all the while eradicating the underlying cause that attracts the infection. When she suggested he meet me and learn what we at Immune Matrix were doing to treat children naturally to resolve chronic ear infections and more importantly prevent stent surgeries in kids, his reply was "my God, she'll put me out of business" (referring to his booked calendar of ear stent operations). He never called to inquire what I had done to help this child avoid surgery and he never referred a child to our clinic to prevent other such surgeries.

This is a sad but common commentary that is so reflective of the dis-incentive doctors have to resolve conditions whenever possible by less intrusive means. Frankly, I look forward to the day when the lack of one or more medical conditions warrants my finding something else to occupy my time with!

Do you want to live like that, without the knowledge or ability to prevent disease? Do you want to live without the knowledge or ability to stop the progression of symptoms that lead you to become prescription drug dependent as the only means to control your symptoms? Do you want to buy into the belief you have no control over whether you can eliminate the cause for your fatigue?

Do you want to buy into the belief only your doctor can help you or he/she has done it all for you already, so you have no recourse but to settle for prescription meds? I certainly hope not. Even with the prescription, do you want to buy into the belief you are married to that prescription "till death do us part" or you cannot improve your health to enable you to reduce or even eliminate your need for that drug?

Can you now see how your perception of low energy affects your choice of a medical practitioner? Do you understand that the thoroughness you will expect from your doctors to come up with answers, not crutches, depends upon you and your doctor sharing the same expectation about energy and vitality?

If you believe low energy is an inevitable fact of aging, then you will be more likely to accept the status quo. You will do very little to be proactive to expect more from your body or your doctor. You will feel powerless and a victim to aging as opposed to someone who sees others around them living active lives despite their increased chronological age. These individuals have their health challenges but they sought answers, persevered and overcame them.

How you perceive what is possible with your energy and health should direct your focus to coming into alignment with likeminded medical practitioners. Becoming aware of your perception and philosophy about energy will enable you to find health care practitioners in alignment with your thinking and goals. It will allow you to quickly identify those who have tuned out, put on blinkers that limit their ability to think outside the "established" allopathic disease paradigm, or don't believe there are any more answers worth seeking.

If you see a doctor that thinks all low energy is due to one cause, for example low thyroid or voices the opinion it's just a normal part of aging, then your options will be limited. Your prospects of reversing and preventing the progressive deterioration and associated low energy decline will be impossible to avert when you align yourself with a doctor with such an attitude.

The challenge you face in finding an experienced medical practitioner, one in sync with your values about health and disease, in sync with your perceptions and expectations that you can improve your energy in many ways goes beyond being dependent upon prescription medication or indefinite supplementation. Your values will make or break your ability to get out of this low energy trap.

Attitude is everything.

Therefore, know your doctor's attitude and aptitude about low energy. This book will help you explore its causes and options. Your health care practitioner should be well versed in everything mentioned in this book. Most are not, which is why this information is offered to you as a navigation and communication tool.

Lastly, the optimal performance of this "invisible" gland I mentioned earlier is vitally important to your mental and physical stamina, immune health, regenerative abilities, mental focus, clarity, and energy biorhythm throughout the day. The health of this "invisible gland" is so important that it should not have to be classified as "diseased" before attention is brought to rebalance and optimize its function. I will discuss it in depth as we proceed.

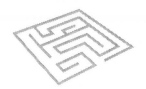

Chapter 5

OBVIOUS LOW ENERGY TRAPS

PART 1 – LIFESTYLE

More and more research confirms lifestyle factors play a significant role in determining what long term conditions we WILL suffer from. Lifestyle habits expose us to certain environmental and nutritional factors that alter our chemistry, metabolism and our genes! Conversely, healthy lifestyle habits can help optimize our health by resetting our metabolism, improving our energy, nutrient absorption, increasing our hormone production, blood circulation and even repairing our genes! Knowing we have the greatest influence over what lifestyle factors we allow ourselves to be affected by should empower us. To know we significantly control our health destiny and can eliminate our symptoms if we learn how to make certain positive changes is truly empowering!

When do we need to take a hard look at our lifestyle? When your lifestyle is such you need a **coping mechanism to maintain function**, then your lifestyle is detrimental to your health. It is at this junction you need to stop and examine your daily habits of living. You need to take a cold objective look at what you are doing, sometimes mindlessly, but daily, to derail your health a little bit at a time. As with termites, the damage they do is largely unseen until a critical mass of damage has occurred. Then the structure begins to fail.

What track are you on?

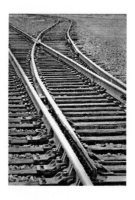

The body is no different. It too becomes eroded by daily bad habits of lifestyle. When you can switch and jump track, things begin to change. However, you need to know what track you are on. Otherwise, your lifestyle might lead you to a place you do not want to go. The scenery may look the same for a time but the destination is not the same. It leads you not to health, but disease. It's the intent of this book to educate and empower you to find answers and get started in reversing the causes for your low energy trap, without surgery and without drugs!

Obvious detrimental lifestyle habits are listed below. They are just the obvious ones and by no means all the things we do to derail our health. When eliminated from your daily habits, your energy will begin to improve like fog lifting from a pond. Your mental focus and stamina will see greater periods of strength like clouds parting in the sky to let in the sunshine. Eliminating bad lifestyle habits will stop sources that tax your body. Your body will once again optimize metabolic, hormone and brain function, essential to break free from your low energy trap.

Do you do any of these?

- skip breakfast
- eat mostly carbohydrates at breakfast, especially refined carbohydrates (cereal, pancakes, bagel, muffin, scones, fruit juice, dairy)

- eat too many carbohydrates at any one meal for your metabolism, resulting in fatigue from progressive insulin resistance
- skip lunch
- eat at irregular times of the day and/or late at night
- wait to eat until your blood sugar has dropped and you are ravenous (going too many hours between meals)
- fail to eat enough protein to maintain steady blood sugar (preferable to eat every 3 hrs. some form of protein with each meal)
- fail to eat sufficient quantities of dark green leafy vegetables
- increase your toxic burden by smoking, drinking alcohol excessively or regularly, eating processed foods, eating canned foods, drinking sodas, recreational drug use
- fail to drink enough water (you need half your weight in ounces daily; 100lb person drinks 50 oz. daily)
- accumulating occupational toxic burdens: car exhaust (truck, bus drivers), chemical exposures (mechanics, dry cleaners, nail salon, industrial chemical plant workers, pesticide applications)
- mold exposures: black mold, or damp/moldy environment, hidden molds in foods (strawberry, grape, raisins, peanut etc.)
- overuse of caffeinated beverages that prevent you from sleeping, and keep you feeling "wired" all day
- snack on sweets, candy, refined carbohydrates for energy pick ups
- get insufficient or no aerobic exercise 3-4 times a week (target heart rate for your age at least 20 minutes duration)
- overuse of computer/TV late into the night preventing you from relaxing and sleeping
- sleep 6 or less hours per night
- have or respond in a stressful way to relationships and work situations
- fail to eat anything green or food with color!
- fail to have at least one bowel movement daily
- fail to sleep in total darkness

- take over the counter medications regularly
- develop nutritional deficiencies from a routine diet, from the regular use of over the counter medications and/or prescription medications
- fail to pay attention to new symptoms or seek medical advise
- fail to maintain a positive outlook on life, negative thinking
- fail to manage the toxic and/or over demanding people in your life

As you can see, what you do daily gives your body the biggest opportunity to help or hinder its maintenance. You might think two martinis or two glasses of wine a day after work to unwind is fine. However, add that up day after day and you have accumulated a huge toxic burden, not to mention the increased metabolic stress imposed from such a lifestyle that you probably haven't compensated for nutritionally. I tell my patients it's what we do "daily" even in small doses that poisons us and derails our health.

PART 2 – THE THYROID

By now you might be thinking, I know why I have low energy, it's my thyroid. It's been that way for years. In fact this problem runs in my family! I've already seen my doctor and I'm on thyroid medication. Sure we've had to change the dose or type of medication but it's being addressed. You think you've done all you can to improve your energy, but you are still in a low energy trap. Do you have to learn to live with it? Not at all!

No matter how long you have had "thyroid issues" and even if you've had to have your thyroid removed, you can still improve your body's usage of thyroid hormones. Even when you cannot manufacture any or enough thyroid hormones, you can still improve your thyroid metabolism.

When we are given thyroid medication to increase our circulating blood levels of thyroid hormone, we hope it helps us to have more energy, among other things. For a while it might feel like the answer. We suddenly feel like our "old" selves. However, over time we seem to regress back into those haunting symptoms of low energy. We go back to our doctor, get more blood tests and are told to stay on the thyroid medication. Our meds may stay the same, change and/or the dosages may increase, but bottom line, we are in a low energy trap despite what we do with our thyroid. So how can we still gain momentum with our thyroid and take a notch out of this low energy trap?

Problem Number One – Blood Levels of Thyroid

Many times we are told our blood levels of thyroid are now "fine" as a result of the thyroid medications our doctor has given us. However, our doctor ignores the question "so why do I still feel so tired?" We are often given the impression that this is all that can be done.

A few times of this round robin with our doctor and we feel we are getting nowhere. We think they've done all they can, all that can be done, and so we begin to believe we need to settle for "this is as good as it gets" level of energy. Not so!

In treating patients with low serum thyroid values in the last dozen years, I have found that most doctors don't test for thyroid antibodies! What does that mean you ask? It means that when your thyroid makes T3 (your thyroid hormone), to put it into simple terms, your immune system creates an antibody and binds to it, preventing your cells from using it! Do these antibodies bind all your T3? No, but if you have a high level of inflammation, your body can develop and/or increase it antibody production to thyroid hormone. Depending upon the level of antibodies produced, some of that hormone will become bound to an antibody and then its usage is unavailable to your cells. You then stay locked in a low energy tap despite adequate levels of thyroid hormone circulating in your blood.

Does the serum T3 test tell my doctor whether I have thyroid antibodies? No. When your doctor orders a blood test for T3, this is the default, the routine test given as part of your CBC panel for standardized blood checkups. This test is automatically done by the lab. It only tests for TOTAL thyroid hormone. What does that mean? Total thyroid hormone means the lab is counting bound (thyroid hormone bound to antibodies) as well as thyroid hormone that is not bound to antibodies.

If your doctor doesn't specifically ask for "FREE T3" to be tested, then the lab automatically tests for "total T3, meaning bound and unbound T3 in your blood. As a result, your blood test results will not be accurate in revealing the level of "available" thyroid hormone you have because it is only the amount of "freeT3" (unbound T3) that determines what is available for your cells to use. The end result is you will get false interpretations from your doctor/labs that show thyroid hormone levels above what your body actually has "free" access too. This is one of the reasons why patients are told their lab values are fine. They may have normal or low normal total T3 levels but in fact be low in free T3!

The irony is that most doctors never test to see if you have thyroid antibodies, and therefore incorrectly assume that when they order "total T3" from the lab, your thyroid hormone levels reflect "free T3" when this is not true. It would be so much more efficient to simply test for Free T3 to ensure an accurate "free" thyroid hormone level if they tested for nothing else. Now that you know this, insist upon having "free" T3 tested every time.

If your free T3 is in the "normal" range, does that mean your thyroid function is normal? Absolutely not! Why can someone take a blood test for thyroid and end up within the normal range and still feel exhausted? There are a few reasons related to how we use our thyroid hormone that will make all the difference in how we feel. This leads us to our next topic, iodine deficiency.

Problem Number Two – Iodine Deficiency

First of all, if we don't have an iodine molecule *attached* to our thyroid hormone cell receptor site, thyroid hormone cannot enter our cell. Take a look at the diagram below. The circle reflects your cell and the "I" is an iodine molecule receptor site. The diagram depicts a cell with two iodine receptor cites. One iodine receptor site has a T3 hormone attached to it. That is where your

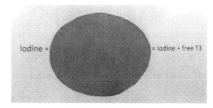

thyroid hormone will be able to enter the cell so that your cell can begin to use it.

If your body is low in iodine, the receptor sites that should have iodine attached, acting like gate keepers, won't. Any receptor site missing iodine prevents your body from using thyroid hormone. Therefore, even though your blood shows adequate amounts of circulating free T3, your cells won't have sufficient access to the hormone for lack of your cell's straw, iodine, to draw thyroid hormone into the cell!

Most of us are low in iodine because the American diet is low in seafood and sea vegetables (seaweed). Iodine infused table salt does NOT provide adequate iodine. In fact, the FDA is contemplating increasing the RDA of iodine from 150mcg daily to 400mcg or more.

Is it simply now a matter of getting more iodine from your diet? Not necessarily. Getting enough iodine to enable your body to use thyroid hormone is a stumbling block not adequately addressed in allopathic medicine. It is largely assumed (incorrectly) if your free T3, if and when it is tested, falls within the normal range, you are considered normal. Nothing could be further from the truth!

Having normal free T3 values doesn't mean you have adequate free T3 entering your cells if your iodine receptor sites lack iodine! In fact, in thirteen years of practice, I have seen too few allopathic physicians who do go the extra route to test for free T3 do anything about assessing whether that patient had sufficient iodine. They certainly know how to test for low iodine, but it just isn't done. It is something that most doctors just doesn't see. This oversight can be a huge clue and answer to helping you out of your low energy trap.

Problem Number Three – Blocked Iodine Receptor Sites!

If iodine deficiency goes largely untested and unseen, consider this monkey wrench on the use of thyroid hormone. Your iodine receptor sites could be blocked! That means something actually takes the place of iodine on the cell receptor site. This in turn prevents your body from taking in your thyroid hormone. It also means what is replacing the iodine molecule on the cell receptor site competes with iodine for that site! What in the world could do that?

A common compound that blocks your iodine receptor sites and directly competes with iodine is bromide! Where is bromide found? It is principally found in refined flour products but is present in other foods as well. Become familiar with where you could be ingesting bromide and eliminate it from your life! You've already been accumulating bromide all your life. However, it's never too late to reduce your current bromide exposure.

To find out more information about the detrimental effects of bromide and how to reduce your exposure check out these online sites:

www.chronicfatigueandnutrition.com
www.breastcancerchoices.org/bromidedominancetheory.html
http://www.acu-cell.com/br.html
http://www.rumormillnews.com/cgi-bin/archive.
cgi?noframes;read=146203

If you stop ingesting bromide containing food will your body eliminate the bromide it has already accumulated? It is not likely, due to the fact that the body stores toxins such as bromide deep in tissue and fat cells when it cannot adequately eliminate them when they were first circulating in the body. Where is bromide stored? Bromide like other toxins can be stored in fat cells, in the matrix between our cells, our connective tissue, muscle, bone and organs. Working with a health care practitioner experienced in "chelation", and the elimination of heavy metals, called "heavy metal chelation" will help you eliminate your toxic burden over time. Bromide is generally eliminated during this process along with heavy metals but it could take more than that to increase your iodine receptor sites to taking in free T3.

There is another way to improve iodine receptor site binding that indirectly eliminates bromide. In the spring of 2012, I attended the Academy of Anti-Aging Conference (A4M) where a study was presented that used 650 mcg per day of iodine to flood the cell receptor sites with iodine. This theoretically knocks off the competing bromide, outnumbering it, allowing for improved usage of thyroid hormone so the presenting doctors conjectured.

Please don't go out and start taking 650mcg of iodine a day without medical supervision as this can cause you to go into too fast of a bromide detoxification. If you have thyroid antibodies and inflammation, taking a sudden large dose of iodine can increase thyroid inflammation. Therefore, begin gradually. There is an accepted protocol for testing one's ability to use thyroid hormone and to monitor one's bromide detoxification that is monitored every two weeks. Therefore, do not do this on your own!

Knowing your morning axillary temperature is an excellent gauge of your thyroid metabolism. Find out. Upon waking take a non-digital thermometer and place it under your armpit for 5 minutes before leaving the bed. Record this reading three days in a row. It will give you an average reading to go by. If it is 97F or below then it suggests you are not using your T3 well and you might either be low in iodine or have blocked iodine receptor sites.

The marker for determining if a patient was improving receptor cite binding of iodine and therefore their use of thyroid hormone was axillary temperature. Most patients with low thyroid hormone usage had axillary (non-digital) temperatures around 95F-97F. I have found this to be true in testing our patients at Immune Matrix. As the level of iodine becomes sustained enough to knock off the competing bromide molecules, more iodine will attach to the cell receptor sites allowing for more thyroid hormone to enter the cell. The result is increased basal metabolic rate as reflected in morning temperature increases. Patients were checked every two weeks. A gradual increase in their axillary temperature also reflected increases in overall energy.

There are also a few astute medical experts up to date on the latest in research in thyroid. Some have published books to educate the public and their colleagues. I highly suggest you read their books if low thyroid has been an issue for you even if you are under regular doctor's care for your thyroid condition:

Why Do I Still Have Thyroid Symptoms? When My Lab Tests Are Normal: A Revolutionary Breakthrough In Understanding Hashimoto's Disease and Hypothyroidism by Datis Kharrazian

and

Thyroid Power by Dr. Richard Shames

Yes it's true. Our nation is facing an epidemic of low thyroid function. Our food, as well as the American diet, is deficient in iodine. Bromide, hidden in food, competes with iodine for those cell receptor sites, blocking what little iodine we can use. Add food sensitivities that cause inflammation, toxic environmental exposure, and you have toxic, inflamed thyroids, with blocked iodine cell receptor sites. Being able to use what little thyroid hormone we make with our fatigued toxic thyroids is a nationwide issue.

Unfortunately, all the components mentioned above, necessary to proper synthesis and use of thyroid hormone, are not routinely addressed in allopathic medicine. The traditional allopathic medical assumption is that if your blood levels of total T3 are within normal range you are using your thyroid hormone adequately. This is absolutely false now that you know we need iodine. The iodine molecule has to be attached to the cell receptor site to enable us to use the hormone, and this hormone cannot be bound to an antibody! Therefore, if your doctor told you your blood work was "fine" for thyroid, and you are still fatigued, you need to find out the details for your lab test. This is what you need to know:

1. Was only total T3 tested? The way to determine what was tested is to look at the lab result. If it shows T3, then it means total T3. This doesn't help you determine how much free and available T3 your cells have access to. You now must return to your doctor and insist that free T3 is tested or find another, more up to date, health care provider to work with.

2. Did the lab test for thyroid antibodies?
    In many cases with routine physicals, only TSH (thyroid stimulating hormone) is tested and nothing else related to the

thyroid. This is a cost saving measure that comes at your expense. There is also a faulty medical assumption at work here. It is presumed if TSH is elevated your body is not making enough thyroid hormone. The body tries to increase the level of TSH to stimulate the manufacture of more T3. However, I routinely see normal TSH levels yet low free T3 levels coupled with low iodine levels. It's entirely inaccurate to base one's medical opinion on how much T3 you make and how well you are able to use it by only testing for TSH. Therefore, if you have had TSH tested but not T3, skip getting tested for T3 and ask that free T3 be tested.

Without the above basic quantifiable information on what your free T3 levels are, you cannot begin to assess how much better your thyroid metabolism could become. Get the right information now.

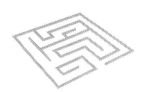

Chapter 6

LESS OBVIOUS LOW ENERGY TRAPS

PART 1 – INSULIN RESISTANCE

A less obvious but equally significant culprit for what could be keeping you in your low energy trap could be directly attributed to the gradual and insidious development of insulin resistance. Just because you don't have diabetes does not mean you are efficient in sugar metabolism. It can still mean you are developing an insulin resistance problem.

Insulin resistance develops when your cells stop responding to the prompts of insulin. When your cells begin to ignore the signal that insulin was designed to prompt (that of allowing simple sugars into the cells where they can be used by the cell), then you begin to develop the condition known as Syndrome X, insulin resistance.

One can be insulin resistant and not have diabetes!

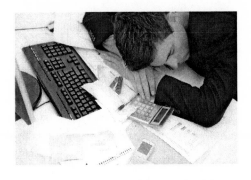

A red flag symptom for insulin resistance is fatigue after eating a meal. It can occur after any meal but is worse with meals containing carbohydrates, especially refined carbohydrates, such as bread or pasta. Fatigue can occur within minutes or be delayed up to an hour or two after a meal. The fatigue can be so bad we have to lie down. We feel totally drained.

As insulin resistance progresses (it depends upon the degree your cells shut off reacting to insulin's signal) your fatigue symptoms also progress in severity. In the beginning, the fatigue feels as if you've had a big meal. We might think we are tired because we are full. That might be the case if you ate a huge meal. However, a large reason for post meal fatigue is you ate more carbohydrates than your body could process. Others might feel a bit slow. With increasing levels of insulin resistance you will find it harder to focus mentally. People often feel they need coffee or some form of caffeine. With more severe insulin resistance you want to close your eyes and take a nap, if only for a few minutes. Some individuals have to nap after meals and that is a very bad sign! There are other signs but fatigue is the easiest barometer to use for our purposes here.

As insulin resistance becomes chronic, the body is less capable of compensating. Your quick pick-ups with caffeine become less effective. Your cells start to ignore small levels of insulin signaling. As a result, the body increases the insulin output. Your cells respond by continuing to ignore the increasing levels of insulin. The post meal fatigue worsens, your fatigue gets drawn out and in some cases over time you become diabetic and a whole new set of metabolic issues arise.

The down side to having your body make too much insulin is akin to your cells crying "wolf". The cells begin to ignore the signal that insulin prompts. The cell shuts off its "sensitivity" to insulin's promptings, ignoring it and in so doing, reducing your ability to process and use carbohydrates and simple sugars. As a result, without cells fed simple sugars necessary for their metabolism, your energy tanks. Your cells will cry out for nutrition and cause you to crave simple sugars, sweets and carbohydrates for quick energy. When you oblige, you feel tired again and the cycle gets worse. Round and round, more insulin resistance is created in a vicious cycle. Therefore, insulin resistance robs your cells of the nutrients they need to create energy in your body. Fatigue is the result, especially after eating carbohydrates.

PART 2 – OTHER CARBOHYDRATE METABOLIC ISSUES

Eating too large a quantity of carbohydrates on a regular basis is a plague of the refined carbohydrate "food in a box" American diet. It is to blame for most of the cases of Syndrome X and insulin resistance. However, other causes besides insulin resistance affect our ability to metabolize complex and simple carbohydrates, preventing us from fully breaking them down.

Immune sensitivities contribute to
the development of insulin resistance.

A less obvious but key reason for challenges with carbohydrate metabolism is the development of **immune sensitivities**. What is an immune sensitivity? Immune sensitivities, as opposed to food allergies, do not show up in standardized allopathic blood tests for "food allergies". An example is to test for a food allergy to oranges. One would have to show positive IgG or IgA antibodies to the phenol in oranges. If you don't have a positive IgG or IgA to orange then it is reported to you that you have no food allergy to orange. Maybe so, but that doesn't mean you won't have "allergy-like" symptoms when you eat the orange! Patients are often told they are not reacting (based upon no positive IgG/IgA antibody responses to food) when in fact they can and are reacting! It is not in their heads.

One can be reactive to oranges, identical to "allergic" symptoms, such as acid reflux or hives from drinking orange juice or any food. Symptoms can include hives, itchy skin, sinus mucous congestion, and scratchy throat. The problem lies in the fact you have developed an immune reaction to a component in the orange such as citric acid, vitamin C, or the bioflavonoids. These components are non-phenol and therefore not considered food allergies but rather food sensitivities. Furthermore, these components, i.e. vitamin C, bioflavonoids and citric acid are not tested in the blood for food allergies!

In the case of your low energy trap, the development and progression of immune sensitivities to various carbohydrates is often the culprit. Foods such as rice, corn, flour, oats, beans, millet, and all sorts of sugars, complex and simple (corn, cane, date, maple, turbinado, fructose, lactose, maltose, honey, & rice syrup) can trigger immune sensitivities that cause allergy-like symptoms.

Food allergies can be easily tested with blood tests. Less accurate is the skin scratch test because the skin has its own immune system. Therefore, the skin can test sensitive to orange when the immune system of the blood/body is not. In addition, the immune system, as reflected in blood tests (IgG, IgA), can change every ninety days as the white blood cells die and either pass on the immune memory or decide not to. The immune memory of the skin stays more or less constant while that of the blood more accurately reflects what is going on with your digestion and body with respect to your overall immune reaction to foods.

Therefore, if you have had a blood test or skin scratch test, you have been tested for allergies but not immune sensitivities. It also means that if you were told that you have no allergy to an orange for example, you might still have a food sensitivity to it. The blood and skin test doesn't diagnose food sensitivities. Bottom line, trust and pay attention to your body's reaction to something.

A diluted immune response will mask "allergic-like" symptoms.

Why is it we often don't know we have a sensitivity to something? It is quite common when we have multiple immune sensitivities to not experience an identifiable symptom directly linked to ingesting that food. This is because the immune response is masked because it has become diluted, akin to being overtaxed. Imagine a balloon that you fill with water. By the same token imagine an immune cell filling up with histamine, the chemical messenger that calls more immune cells to the location where histamine is released. Histamine serves to attract more immune cells to deal with what the immune system perceives as an infection, something foreign (like undigested food, chemicals), or something not handled well by the body, such as a toxin.

If your water balloon is full of water and you have one target, you can drench your target with a lot of water from your balloon. However, if you have 25 targets, you are only able to splash a bit of water on each target with some getting more water, some getting less. The same goes for the immune cell. If your immune cell recognizes 25 allergens, then the amount of histamine it has to target each allergen is smaller. That means you have a smaller immune response per allergen because you have less histamine associated with that allergen. It may therefore appear to you that you don't have food sensitivities because when you eat that orange you either don't notice a reaction, or the reaction is so mild you don't associate it with an allergy-type reaction! The more histamine released, the greater the immune response. When the quantity of histamine released per antigen is small, so is the immune response to that antigen. But the cumulative effect of small amounts of histamine on 25 subjects can take a global toll on the body. That is why fatigue after eating food can either be a sign of insulin resistance or food sensitivities or both!

In summary therefore, when eating a food, the immune trigger can be the phenol in the food (making it a food allergy) or a component in the food (making it a food sensitivity) for which the symptoms can be the same. Anyone can develop and suffer from immune sensitivities to anything they eat: carbohydrates, proteins, fats, fiber, acids, vitamins, minerals, food additives, preservatives, colorings, synthetic vitamins and their additives. The list is nearly endless! Corn sugar, malt (the sugar in gluten), lactose, beet sugar, fructose (fruit sugar), and honey are common food sensitivities to carbohydrates that lead to the development of insulin resistance. With insulin resistance comes more metabolic fatigue and the development of more food, chemical and environmental sensitivities. It becomes a slow downward spiral that will keep you metabolically locked in your low energy trap.

PART 3 – IMMUNE BASED NUTRIENT DEFICIENCIES

Nutrient deficiencies can keep you in your low energy trap. You can develop nutrient deficiencies from a habitual diet lacking in certain nutrients your body needs. A common example is the classic American diet high in refined carbohydrates and low in dark green leafy vegetables that are otherwise high in alkaline minerals. As I mentioned previously, carbohydrates cause our body to become acidic, burning up our alkaline mineral stores faster. If you also rarely or never eat dark green leafy vegetables, your ability to replenish your alkaline mineral reserves is low. As a result you can begin to develop fatigue from specific nutrient deficiencies associated with low B12, B6, magnesium, zinc, trace minerals, chromium, selenium, molybdenum and many other core nutrients. The imbalanced diet causes your nutrient deficiency because the imbalance makes you "high octane" per say for core nutrients that would neutralize the damaging effects of your imbalanced diet. Persistent nutrient deficiency from an imbalanced diet locks you in your low energy trap!

An imbalanced diet can cause nutrient deficiencies.

You can also become deficient in the very nutrient you have developed an immune sensitivity to because the immune system can block its use. The immune system, once triggered to recognize something sees that nutrient as a foreign entity and deals with it accordingly. You can become deficient in any nutrient when this occurs. Bioflavonoids, citric acid, certain amino acids such as methionine (the key amino acid needed by the liver to detoxify), vitamin B, C, E, magnesium, calcium, B12, folate, zinc, and copper are common culprits of immune attack that lead to deficiencies in these nutrients, keeping you in your low energy trap directly or indirectly.

Your immune system can block nutrient
absorption, causing nutrient deficiencies.

The nutrient deficiency isn't necessarily due to lack of consumption of these nutrients. Many patients naturally avoid the foods they are sensitive too, such as orange juice. The deficiency can be a byproduct of one's immune interference with its metabolism. Most doctors don't suspect this as their first reaction but rather assume that you are not ingesting enough of this nutrient. When your lab results come back and you are low in a nutrient their first impulse is to tell you to get more of this nutrient or they prescribe a supplement for this deficiency. This is an all too common practice in treating autism.

When your immune system has blocked the break down and processing of a nutrient, elevated levels can circulate in the blood giving a false high, or the patient may test for low nutrient levels when excretions are not hindered by the immune system. Hidden immune sensitivities to nutrients affect one's break down, absorption and excretion of a nutrient. When the patient is then told to eat more or take more of the specific nutrient, they often suffer symptoms. This is because immune system causes inflammation when you eat it. But eating it still keeps you in a state of nutrient deficiency. Taking more of this nutrient only fuels the fire of immune reaction, increasing your overall inflammation. As a result, many individuals will not feel good on certain supplements. Immune system interference with metabolism is often the silent culprit!

When you do try to take a supplement to increase your vitamin C or bioflavonoids, for example, you feel lousy from it and stop taking it. That is because you have developed an immune sensitivity to it. This cannot be detected in food allergy testing! Taking more only causes more immune inflammation and inflammatory symptoms in direct proportion to the amount you ingest. This is why in some patients with allergies, as in the case of autism, taking more B vitamins may not increase their serum levels of the vitamin. They will feel lousy and some even have aggressive behavior in reaction to taking it, all because it triggers immune inflammation from taking the supplement.

I have treated many autistic patients already on "DAN" protocols (Defeat Autism Now Protocols) or other treatment programs who were instructed to use focused intensive vitamin therapy for nutrient deficiencies as revealed in their lab tests. Some of these children literally "flunk" out of the protocol because they gradually react to the supplements given until they can no longer tolerate them. I have found this happens because their immune system has developed an immune sensitivity to the very supplement they were taking. We at Immune Matrix have a proprietary and holistic way of reversing that immune recognition allowing the patient to reduce their inflammatory load and begin to digest and absorb their nutrients again.

Immune sensitivities can alter carbohydrate metabolism.

Chronic inflammatory disorders often cause challenges in breaking down carbohydrates into simple sugars. Many such patients I test are found to have developed immune sensitivities to simple sugars such as fructose, lactose, malt, beet, corn, turbinado, cane sugar, and even honey. In addition, those individuals with known digestive issues such as acid reflux, irritable bowel or skin disorders such as eczema, all commonly have some degree of food sensitivities for which simple sugars are the most common.

The more inflammation, the more likely fatigue is one of the symptoms. Now you know one more cause that is keeping you in your low energy trap! Why is that? Having developed immune sensitivities to carbohydrates limits the efficiency the body has in digesting (aka breaking down complex carbohydrates i.e. the potato, an apple, or glass of milk, into simple sugars such as glucose, fructose and/or lactose) and using those individual components for cellular function. When your digestion does not adequately break down a complex carbohydrate into its simple sugar components, the cell goes hungry. Why? Because only the simple sugar molecule is small enough to fit into the cell membrane's receptor site, enabling it to enter the cell like lock and key. Unless the simple sugar, such as fructose can enter the cell, the cell is unable to use that sugar for energy. The result is you will feel tired! You will also be sent a signal from the cell to eat more carbs! The cell wants to be fed!

Take a look at the diagram below. At the top of the cell you see "undigested sugar" and it is reflected in a large carbohydrate molecule depicted as g-g-g-g. The simple sugar used here is glucose and when it is available in that form it easily passes through the cell receptor site and is able to "feed" the cell, giving you energy.

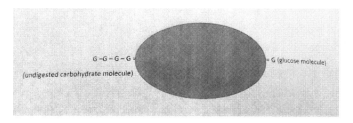

What happens when your cells are not being fed because your digestion is not breaking down your carbohydrates into simple sugars? Your cell sends out a hormonal signal to increase your body's insulin production. Insulin helps the cell to take in and absorb simple sugars. The cell doesn't know that the problem isn't with the "escort molecule" insulin but with the availability of adequately broken down simple sugars to actually be absorbed. Without enough simple sugars to feed your cells, all the insulin in the world won't help those cells to suck in those simple sugars. The end result over time is that the cell begins to ignore the insulin signal. The body then tries to increase the volume of that signal by increasing the amount of insulin secreted. The cells continue to ignore aka resist the signal. This leads to insulin resistance as the body pumps out more insulin in a vain attempt to increase absorption of simple sugars to feed the cells.

When you eat more carbohydrates than your body can break down and absorb, or if you eat certain carbohydrates that your body is struggling to break down (due to immune sensitivies, lack of digestive enzymes or problems with leaky gut), then you will create insulin resistance. This problem will get worse over time.

What the body doesn't realize is that the problem isn't a deficiency of insulin output; it's more a matter of basic simple sugar building blocks of nutrition not having been broken down small enough to allow the cells to absorb them. Without the insulin you don't have the transport of simple sugars across the cell wall into the cell. You need the simple sugars to be broken down and ready for transport. Without that happening your cells will crank up the insulin signal in a desperate attempt to pull in the sugars they need.

Inadequate digestion keeps you locked in low energy.

What happens when your digestion is unable to break down food to its simple amino acid, fatty acid and simple sugar components? Cellular malnutrition occurs. When the lack of break down is carbohydrates, you will develop insulin resistance. This cellular malnutrition causes your body to respond with fatigue, sugar cravings and increased insulin output, all in a vain attempt to get those nutrients into the cells. Rather than cellular nutrition, your body's attempt to compensate pushes you deeper into insulin resistance, cyclical fatigue or worse, diabetes. All the while your energy wanes and you stay trapped in an unending cycle of low energy.

Other culprits besides the inefficient break down of carbohydrates leading to insulin resistance are:

- immune sensitivities to many carbohydrates such as corn, oat, gluten, and rice, potato
- low production of digestive enzymes needed to break down these carbohydrates into their simple sugars
- leaky gut (which causes undigested carbohydrates (large molecules) to pass into the bloodstream) triggering the immune system to see these large molecules as foreign, thus the development of immune sensitivities to the very foods you can't digest well

The eventual progression and worsening of carbohydrate metabolism, food sensitivities and insulin resistance will stress what I will call your "invisible" gland. I call it "invisible" in this book to get my point across that this gland is largely overlooked by most systems of medicine. This gland is not given the credit it deserves for the role it plays in contributing to the development of insulin resistance, immune weakness and chronic fatigue. Before we speak of this gland let's look at other causes for your low energy trap.

PART 4 – CHRONIC HIDDEN VIRAL INFECTION

Undetected chronic viral infection is very common. Like holding a beach ball under water, the effort the body has to make to control the life cycle of the viruses that have invaded it is a constant 24/7. This fatigues the immune system over time as it is not meant to be under constant siege. Stress and imbalanced nutritional factors, especially those that can make viral replication favorable as with L-lycine and B vitamin deficiencies, renders the body ineffective in suppressing the expression of the virus. Symptoms may then begin to manifest sporadically or cyclically depending upon the virus and how it manifests in the body.

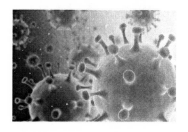

A common insidious feature of viruses is low energy! They may cause cyclical low energy, the type you feel after not having had enough rest or sleep. They may cause a type of low energy that comes from over exertion but now lasts well past when you should have recovered from your exertion. This can be a symptom of viral involvement. You could even suffer a type of low energy that makes you feel like you will never feel like your old self again to live and do things you once enjoyed without a second thought.

There are many types of chronic viral infections. A common culprit involves 25 known strains of the herpes family alone, they include:

Herpes simplex virus Type 1 (HSV-1)
Herpes simplex virus Type 2 (HSV-2)
Epstein Barr virus (EBV)
Cytomegalovirus (CMV)
Varicella Zoster Virus (VZV)
Human herpes virus 6 (HHV family)
(exanthum subitum or roseola infantum)
Human herpes virus 8 (Kaposi's sarcoma-associated herpes virus)

Not all of these viruses cause chronic fatigue in and of themselves. We can harbor more than one type of virus. Cumulatively, they wear down the immune system and keep us in our low energy trap. Add their effect to the cumulative effect of other low grade and often hidden infections (as in hidden bacterial infection in the gums and gut) and you have a recipe for chronic fatigue. Together they dilute the effort of your immune cells. It's like having an army under attack not from one enemy but several groups of enemies. Eventually one's energy, vitality and mortality will be affected.

Chronic viral infections can be mild enough (as in that water balloon example) that we have no idea we carry them! Our immune response to them is so diluted to all the things our immune system is reactive to, we become unaware of our body's effort to fight them. Instead, we may blame our lack of energy on something entirely different:

- diagnosed low thyroid hormone output
- insulin resistance
- sleep issues
- being out of shape
- being overstressed
- having another condition such as Lyme disease or allergies or another immune based disorder
- allergies or immune sensitivities
- a nutrient deficiency
- a diagnosed disease (blaming it all on that one thing)
- the effects of aging

Viruses contribute to cyclical fatigue.

These viruses can impact thyroid function, causing its function to decline. Unless the viral count in your body is reduced or eliminated, your thyroid can never recover. You will then be required to be on thyroid medications indefinitely! Whether you have one family of virus or multiple, they collectively contribute to cyclical fatigue. Therefore, they will play a significant role in keeping you in your low energy trap.

Sadly, most allopathic doctors do not look to the cause or trigger for why the thyroid function has declined because the prevailing attitude is that you can survive on your crutch, thyroid meds for life. Is that how you want to live, without the prospect of regaining some or all of your thyroid function without medication?

What if these viruses affect other organs? They are known to affect other glands and organs: parotid, parathyroid, brain, heart and that "invisible" gland! If these organs and glands are attacked, you will see cyclical issues with these organs, an overall decline of organ function and fatigue that keeps you in that low energy trap like a prison.

Chronic fatigue viruses such as Epstein Barr, cytomegalovirus and echo virus hit you like the flu initially. One does not have to be taken out by the virus, as in the case with "mono", to suffer long standing recurrent bouts of fatigue caused by one of these viruses. The only difference is that after you recover from what you think is the flu; you never regain your "old" energy back. You begin to suffer bouts of recurrent fatigue, especially when stressed. Your ability to rebound from stress and activity diminish more and more. The severity varies from mild to intermittent, getting progressively debilitating, and then chronic. You may go on to develop low thyroid function and other organ symptoms.

In addition, Epstein Bar, the biggest culprit in cyclical fatigue, can and often does attack the thyroid and parathyroid glands. It weakens them causing suboptimal thyroid hormone production. This virus also crosses the blood-brain barrier to enter the brain. It is known to contribute to the formation of certain cancers, including that of the brain (there are different forms of brain cancer). I have also seen in certain individuals with high viral counts more symptoms associated with brain inflammation: trouble with focus and concentration, decreased desire to read, trouble concentrating and staying on task, as well as short term memory lapses.

I have yet to find a patient of mine (who has tested positive for Epstein Bar) receive any other advise by their allopathic doctor other than to go home and rest. What is more alarming is that I have had many such patients receive the comment from their allopathic doctors that "everyone is exposed to this virus, it's no big deal to have it". Considering that this virus is a huge culprit in weakening one's energy, glands, and causing chronic inflammation in the brain and other tissues, the fact that allopathic medicine does not have a "drug" to treat it is no reason to placate its significance in contributing to the low energy trap!

In fact, research as long as five years ago already established the exact mechanism whereby proteins from the Epstein Bar virus known as EBNA1 cause the progressive loss of protective proteins of the body called PML nuclear bodies. Once these nuclear bodies are damaged, tumors and cancer are allowed to flourish. Sivachandran N, Sarkari F, Frappier L. Epstein-Barr Nuclear Antigen 1 Contributes to Nasopharyngeal Carcinoma through Disruption of PML Nuclear Bodies. *PLoS Pathog*, 4(10): e1000170 DOI: 10.1371/journal.ppat.1000170

What happens in the case of chronic low grade brain inflammation? You think your brain is getting old. You have brain fog (foggy or slower processing), problems maintaining sustained levels of focus and concentration, lowered brain stamina and challenges with maintaining your quick sharp mental reactive responses. You might go on to develop recurrent headaches or migraines. Your pre-existing headaches or migraines become more frequent and severe and don't respond to the medications that use to work for you! You might begin to feel your brain is making the rest of your body tired, leading to whole body fatigue intermittently, sustained low grade, or cyclically.

Most individuals have no idea they harbor the Epstein Bar virus.

With many patients, their doctors have no idea they suffer from the effects of chronic Epstein Bar. Unless the case is acute (meaning recently acquired) and you present with severe flu like symptoms, your doctor has no idea you are harboring this virus. Even then, a common flu is often to blame. Your doctor would have to be psychic to guess that Epstein Bar is a culprit in your chronic low energy picture. We, at Immune Matrix clinics have a proprietary way of testing our patient's immune response to the virus. When weakened, it's a red flag that there has not only been an exposure but the immune system is fatigued to fighting the virus. In such case we order labs to confirm our findings and treat the patient to lower their viral count.

If you are the least suspicious you might harbor this virus, you can have a viral titer (called a DNA quant) ordered by your doctor. Getting a viral titer means the lab does a count of the amount of viral proteins circulating in your bloodstream. It's a fail proof way to determine your viral load, as opposed to antibody titers. The standard practice is to test for antibodies to the virus, but this does not tell us how virulent the virus is in your system especially if your immune system is fatigued.

Your viral antibody titers could show a false low when your immune system is fatigued to the virus because your body will not be able to make sufficient quantities of antibodies. When a low antibody count is found, it is assumed by allopathic medicine that you have not been exposed or that you don't have the pathogen. This is often an incorrect assumption. If your body has been fighting this pathogen for a long time, and your immune defenses become fatigued, your body can fail to make sufficient amount of antibodies. Thus a low antibody count, or a zero antibody count could be a false low while your body is under siege with high levels of the virus!

Your viral count could actually be very high though your antibody count is zero to low. Finding your viral load will tell you how well your immune system is dealing with the virus, or not! Don't get lulled into being told by your doctor that since your antibody count to the virus is low or even non-existent, you don't have the virus or you don't have a significant level of this virus in your system. I see this false assumption occurring frequently with my own patients. They test negative to antibodies to certain viruses and are wrongly told they have no exposure to the virus as a result. When we boost their immune system function and get a viral DNA quant, we find very high levels of the virus in their system.

In most cases you will have to insist on the "DNA quant" test with your doctor and not settle for antibody tests alone. Ask for a "viral titer" or "DNA quant". Your doctor will know what to write down on the lab requisition form. This way you will know the potency of the virus in your system (the amount of viral DNA) and be able to determine if any treatment protocol drops the viral count. This is exactly how I monitor the effectiveness of our treatment protocols for Epstein Bar. This virus is getting harder and harder to fight! I've seen significant changes in the last two years with patients where it is taking longer and longer to drop the viral count. Now it's nearly impossible to eradicate, especially in those patients suffering from Lyme pathogens (there are over 300 types of Lyme disease associated pathogens).

If you do have a high viral load, don't let your doctor downplay it by saying everyone has it. Use the viral DNA quant test to gauge the effectiveness of any anti-viral protocols based upon how well they bring down your viral load. You could very well see your thyroid function and your energy improve in addition to mental clarity and stamina. You will also ward off the future development of tumors and possibly cancer!

Get a DNA quant.

The total elimination of two other viruses that could be keeping you in your low energy trap, echo and cytomegalovirus, is still possible. These can also be identified by viral titers. However, bear in mind that allopathic medicine is weakest in the treatment of viral infection, chronic inflammation and immune disorders. Their tool box per se historically has been limited to the development of anti-virals (viral suppressing drugs) in the Herpes family. As a result, taking prescription anti-viral drugs has been the classic way to "suppress" a herpes virus but not viruses outside this family.

I have seen some doctors give their patients the same herpes anti-viral drugs for the long term management of Epstein Bar. However, in treating patients with chronic inflammation, immune sensitivities, and chronic viral infections, I have found those patients that refrain from taking prescription anti-viral drugs while on specific treatment protocols designed to kill and excrete the virus were more successful in reducing and eliminating viral titers for Epstein Bar than those simultaneously taking the prescription anti-viral. I am not sure the reason why, but it's as if the immune system has to have open season on being able to fight the virus without the interference of the anti-viral drug's effect upon the replication of the virus. More investigation is warranted.

Clinical research is under way to find other natural anti-microbial agents that will effectively eliminate the Epstein Bar viral load. Promising horizons are opening up for the use of essential oils, vitamin K and potent anti-microbial plant based extracts to help fight viral and Lyme co-infectants. Immune Matrix is currently investigating the use of such nutrients and essential oils and has had some surprising and promising outcomes! Further research and investigation is certainly needed.

PART 5 – CHRONIC HIDDEN BACTERIAL INFECTION

Chronic hidden bacterial infection that keeps you in your low energy trap can be found in two main locations. One type lives in your colon as "dysbiotic" bacteria. These bacteria are not considered "normal" gut flora. That is why they are called dysbiotic. In an effort to set up house in your digestive system, they attach to the lining of your intestines and in so doing create microscopic holes. As you digest your food, various degrees of undigested food will leak through these holes and enter the blood stream and lymphatic system where your immune system will become triggered to see these undigested food particles as foreign proteins. These undigested food particles now infiltrating your blood and lymphatic system will prompt the development of food sensitivities and inflammatory disorders. This is how dysbiotic bacteria lead to the formation of leaky gut and the eventual development of food sensitivities.

Bacteria located in the gums are another major source of infection for the entire body. Bacteria lodged in your gums creates gum inflammation. These bacteria lead to gum irritation, teeth and gum sensitivity and gingivitis. You can have chronic gum inflammation and not be aware of it!

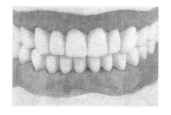

The bacteria circulate in your saliva and drain down the lymphatic system in your neck. There they end up deposited in your digestive tract. This is how we can develop dysbiosis even when we take probiotics and/ or eat cultured vegetables. These pathogens continually circulate in your bloodstream. They also circulate in your saliva, are swallowed and can implant and grow in your colon and become dysbiotic flora! This is why good gum health is essential! Otherwise, you are contaminating your entire body with bacteria. It is well noted in medicine that gum health is directly proportional to longevity. The more infected the gums, the shorter the life span.

Like a rain, your immune system has to fight off and prevent the takeover of these bacteria as they rain down upon your organs. In most healthy individuals, these bacteria will simply crowd out the probiotic flora. Probiotic flora produce B12 and other cofactors necessary to make energy and assist in detoxification. Dysbiotic bacteria will not do this. The bacteria hidden in your digestive track and gums circulate and bathe your organs and glands with bacteria. These bacteria will also cause leaky gut and food sensitivities over time. They can in turn recolonize in joints leading to chronic joint inflammation and the need for joint replacement, brain inflammation, connective tissue weakness, degeneration and inflammation, heart valve erosion, inflammation of the lining of arteries, veins, capillaries leading to plaque formation (atherosclerosis) and hardening of the arteries (arteriosclerosis). The effects of hidden bacterial infection are a leading silent killer in America!

If your gums keep "seeding" the digestive tract via the lymphatic fluids, then some of these bacteria from your gums will end up living in your digestive tract. Others will circulate in your bloodstream and cause joint pain. Others still will inflame the arteries, veins and capillaries as they circulate in your blood vessels and cause atherosclerosis (silent thickening of the plaque in your circulatory system, eventually leading to arteriosclerosis, the hardening of your circulatory system). Some bacteria, as they drain down through the lymphatic system in your neck will bathe your thyroid gland with bacteria laden fluid. Is it no wonder why your thyroid hasn't been working well for so long?

Stop the bacteria rain!

Bacteria also hide out in the wisdom tooth pockets. This is the area left in the gum/bone after the wisdom tooth is pulled out. Long after the wisdom tooth has been extracted, bacteria set up house. They are mostly silent in terms of symptoms. They don't generally cause symptoms because they are so low grade. Immune Matrix screens their patients' teeth and has found that Lyme pathogens love to live in the wisdom pockets! To some degree this makes sense as Lyme pathogens are known to gravitate to sites of trauma. Tooth extraction is trauma. Therefore, bad gums aka gingivitis, can and do contribute to your having dysbiosis and leaky gut. This in turn leads to food allergies, fatigue and chronic inflammatory symptoms. When Lyme pathogens reside in wisdom pockets, this too becomes a focal point of circulation for Lyme pathogens for the entire body through your saliva.

What can we do about these so called silent gum inflammations? Some state of the art biological dentists use ozone to inject the gums and wisdom pockets. Immune Matrix checks its patients suffering from Lyme disease and those with chronic dysbiosis and infection to determine if they need ozone injections. This helps to eliminate another source of why the colon is colonized with dysbiotic bacteria and the recirculation of Lyme pathogens. Simply eliminating dysbiotic bacteria from the colon doesn't necessarily mean that bacteria will not recolonize in it again if your gums & wisdom pockets have been ignored!

These circulating bacteria can also attack and weaken your glands, kidneys, thyroid, parathyroid as well as that "silent" gland I have yet to speak of. Their constant presence around and in your glandular tissue prevents their optimal performance, keeping you in your low energy trap. They will also hinder the optimal performance of your digestive tract preventing complete breakdown of your food. Their constant presence in your body can cause systemic (whole body) inflammation (joints, tendons, muscles, connective tissue) which hinders the effectiveness of your body's ability to fight infection. Remember the example of the army with too many enemy groups to fight? The same goes for your immune system. Its effectiveness is diluted in direct proportion to the number and volume of immune triggers it has to deal with. As a result, the body becomes run down, like a fence in disrepair, weakened from wear and tear. The same result can occur with your tissues.

These bacteria, once they attack your glands, cause poor glandular performance. The result is lower hormone production leading to fatigue. Lyme co-infectants such as Babesia, Bartonella, and a few hundred other species of bacteria and spirochetes can also weaken glands. Their presence in the wisdom pockets can be a constant source of pathogenic rain to the body.

Immune Matrix identifies those patients with positive gum and wisdom tooth signatures and refers them to biological dentists for ozone injections. Generally, within two ozone injection sessions, the localized infiltration is eliminated and the systemic rain of bacteria that stresses the organs and glands is eliminated. This can greatly help in the fight against chronic Lyme disease if only it were regularly tested and treated. It can also significantly aid in regaining one's thyroid function by eliminating the constant pathogenic rain.

This pathogenic rain can also weaken one's immune system. The constant effort to regenerate immune cells to keep up with the pathogenic load, leads to fatigue. I tell my patients this example frequently. Imagine keeping a beach ball under water with one hand. It takes constant effort. As soon as you let up the pressure on your hand, the ball pops up. Imagine the beach ball as the pathogen and your hand as the immune system. That is how viruses and bacteria work in your body when your immune system fatigues in its effort to combat persistent infection. Over time, the immune system can and does fatigue to the constant presence of pathogens.

Your immune system must recognize the pathogen to have any hope of eliminating or controlling it.

Immune cells are called to the site of inflammation, trauma or infection by chemical signals, such as the histamine example mentioned earlier. However, calling an immune cell to the site of infection is not a guarantee that it will in fact kill the pathogen. The immune system must be able to recognize the pathogen and have sufficient "soldiers" to fight the battle with or without the added "ammunition" of the antibiotic or antifungal medication. This explains in part why simply taking an antibiotic for bacterial infection or an anti-fungal for yeast/mold/candida infection can be ineffective. Your immune system has to recognize the enemy to fight it. All the ammunition in the world will not prompt it to kill the enemy when it doesn't realize it has a real enemy to kill. This is often the culprit when patients have to take antibiotics or antifungals for a long period of time. I'm referring to taking these medications for weeks on end. In the Lyme disease community patients are often given such drugs for years continuously! Once we boost immune recognition to the pathogen, we stop this cycle of long term ineffective medication. Similar situations occur with cystic acne. The body fatigues to the systemic bacterial infection which is one reason the patient has to take antibiotics repetitively or consistently.

Since your immune system must work 24/7 to detect and kill pathogens, it can and will fatigue to the ever present pressure of pathogens constantly seeking to multiply and thrive inside your body. New white blood cells (a component of your immune system) are born and raised up to "recognize" the enemy. This immune memory is passed on from the expiring white blood cell. The life cycle of the white blood cell turns over every ninety days. Sometimes, this is not fast enough to compete with the life cycle of some pathogens, especially if the stress to the immune system has been constant. This is when essential components in bone marrow necessary to make new white blood cells can become depleted, slowing the production of new baby white blood cells. The end result is your organs and other metabolic systems operate under a state of constant low grade inflammation. This leads to a lack of tissue repair and regeneration. The result is suboptimal tissue/gland/organ function and nutrient malabsorption, a guarantee that you will stay locked in your low energy trap.

When pathogens outnumber the immune system and gain an upper hand in your body, especially when the demand for constant synthesis of new immune cells taxes the body's ability to keep up with the production needs of the immune system, then and only then will you see symptoms from the pathogens manifest. Such symptoms include but are not limited to fatigue, joint pain, slow recovery from exertion, and brain fog/fatigue to name a few. Your tissues degenerate when the body cannot keep up with repair. Muscle weakness, muscle aches, muscle fatigue, in addition to organ and brain fatigue can result.

Immune Matrix measures the relative degree of inflammation and degenerative state of tissues by monitoring a patient's BIA (bioelectrical impedance analysis) as part of their treatment protocol. Electrodes are attached to one hand and foot on one side of the body. The BIA machine takes specific measurements that can be used as markers for dehydration, toxic retention, and many other vital parameters. It is particularly useful in helping Immune Matrix to monitor their patients' hydration, toxic retention and regenerative abilities. Furthermore, the BIA helps us to assess the effectiveness or non-effectiveness of any supplement/medication protocol by quantifying certain health parameters. This is especially important when aggressive antibiotic therapy is used long term, as in the case of many Lyme disease treatment protocols. This type of testing becomes crucial in assessing whether the treatment is causing undue and accelerated degeneration of tissues.

Tissue degeneration is unavoidable with any long term inflammatory illnesses. However, a treatment protocol can unknowingly exact a high toll on tissues if not caught. Knowing when to take a break from treatment to help the body detoxify and rid itself of pathogen die-off and focus on regeneration is a little appreciated but essential component of healing that Immune Matrix is passionate about educating doctors and patients alike suffering from chronic infectious disorders.

BIA monitoring thus becomes an invaluable assessment tool to determine if symptoms are due to the suspected pathogen itself or derive from the side-effects (degenerative/toxic accumulation) of treatment, or a combination of both. The quantifiable data gained from regular BIA testing helps the trained practitioner to assess a patient's progress in reducing inflammation, toxic retention and load, detoxification efficiency, nutrient absorption and tissue repair.

The BIA test results help us to confirm that the patient is on the mend so to speak as opposed to folding under ever increasing degrees of inflammation from die-off, or increased toxic retention. Without the benefit of this technology to assist us in monitoring bio-markers of health, much in the way of chronic inflammation and infection would go undetected or worse, symptoms would be erroneously attributed to something non-causative.

This oversight by medical practitioners, even specialists in Lyme disease treatment occurs more than you can imagine. In fact, it is not the norm to quantify a patient's progress and thus the room for error is huge! The result often is over medication and extended prescription drug and herbal treatment well beyond what the body can handle. The patient becomes progressively worse. All the while the doctor thinks the pathogen is to blame. In fact, what is really happening in many cases is the patient's body has not been able to keep up with the fall-out from the treatment to cleanse and regenerate tissue. Chronic candidiasis, leaky gut, hidden streptococcus infection, dehydration and malabsorption have all been mistaken for the original diagnosed infection that was presumed the primary cause. Sadly, this happens regularly!

You might ask "Wouldn't I know if I had a chronic infection? Nope. These chronic pathogens will not generally cause sudden fevers or symptoms that make you sit up and take notice you have an infection as they would when you initially contracted them. This is why their presence is more nefarious and subtle, like having termites! You don't get obvious symptoms something is wrong until the damage is extensive.

These pathogens are stealthy. They want to set up house inside of you. Therefore, they learn how to evade detection to thrive inside of you without killing you! As your immune system becomes less resilient with their persistent presence (like keeping that beach ball under water), you are less and less able to recover your energy, your metabolic function and repair tissue. You experience more cyclical fatigue and degenerative function.

Your immune cells can begin to habituate to and stop eradicating the pathogen. Other immune cells fatigue to their presence and seemingly ignore some of the pathogens for lack of immune recognition and/or function. This allows the pathogens to grow and flourish inside your tissues and impede the function of your organs ever so slightly. The result is gradual and cyclical bouts of low energy.

We have found in treating patients suffering from chronic infection at Immune Matrix clinics, boosting immune recognition (through our Immune Reset™ protocol) to the specific pathogen the immune system tested ineffective against, therapies previously ineffective now became effective. This is how our Immune Reset™ protocol came into being.

A great cure is akin to having a great tennis racket, but can your body use it well?

The focus in allopathic medicine is to have a great cure. That is akin to having a great tennis racket or golf club. It presumes however that your body is a great tennis player or golfer! If your body were somehow out of shape, or totally incapable of swinging that racket or golf club, then the best piece of equipment will do little to improve your game. The same is true for medications and supplements. Having a great remedy does very little to eradicate a pathogen when the immune system doesn't recognize the pathogen or blocks the use of the medication or supplement because it has become sensitized to it.

This is why so many products, no matter how expensive, will work for one person but not another, especially those suffering from long term inflammatory conditions. How many of you know of someone that gets sick or feels bad from taking a vitamin, supplement or medication? Their immune system has come to (generally via leaky gut) recognize the undigested medication or supplement and cause the body to react to it. This is the common reason in most cases. Immune Matrix helps to identify these situations and through our treatment protocols, reverse the inappropriate immune reaction, thereby optimizing nutrient and medicine usage.

Sometimes the immune system stops recognizing a pathogen because of immune system "fatigue". The exact causes are multiple. The end effect is akin to giving a five year old an assault rifle and telling them to shoot the enemy. They don't know who it is and will kill the wrong person as a result.

This is one mechanism how the immune system can inadvertently cause damage to our own tissue in an attempt to also eradicate the pathogens by recognizing thyroid, joint, and/or tendon tissue and more. It is also a key mechanism for how hidden chronic infections can lead to low energy and cyclical fatigue.

Besides fatigue, do hidden bacterial infections pose any other threat to our health? Hidden bacteria pathogens commonly lead to degenerative conditions such as arteriosclerosis, erosion of heart valves, phlebitis, and hip replacements. They lead to chronic inflammatory disorders such as arthritis, cystitis, food sensitivities, skin disorders and eruptions, eczema, and irritable bladder. They lead to chronic gut dysbiosis which causes bloating, constipation and/or diarrhea, leaky gut and irritable bowel. They can also cause acid reflux, headache, migraine, itchy and/or painful ears, chronic ear and sinus infections and once inside the brain, any type of brain fog, auditory or verbal processing issues, including headache and/or migraine. This is especially suspect in those patients that do not respond well to classical migraine medications. These individuals often had a history of childhood ear infections that were severe or repetitive. The bacteria can cross the thin temporal bones and enter the brain where they cause low grade brain inflammation leading to developmental brain function disorders and cyclical headaches and migraine.

If you wait long enough, a hip or heart valve replacement might be necessary. Then you will surely need your allopathic physician. But why wait until you get such a diagnosis? If you are not diligent in seeking answers to subtle symptoms that impact your energy and lifestyle now, waiting will surely see you in a doctor's office with a "disease" diagnosis that could have been averted years earlier.

Acknowledgement and recognition that symptoms from bacterial infections often run silent is neglected in the face of other more glaring and pressing symptoms in allopathic medicine. Acknowledging and addressing the effects these hidden bacterial infections have upon organ function, prior to a disease diagnoses and the development of other more chronic organ pathologies, is not a focus unless the doctor is trained in functional medicine and has a keen understanding of chronic inflammation and its signs (despite their limited tools to deal with them by prescription drug protocols). More and more doctors are learning about herbal remedies and combined drainage/homeopathic formulas. Many refer out/or are beginning to incorporate them into their practice. We often see greater effectiveness in outcomes due to the reduced likelihood of pathogen resistance and improved excretion of microbial metabolites (die-off). However, these pioneering allopathic doctors are still a minority.

Many chronic bacterial infections harbor drug resistant strains such as alpha, beta and gamma streptococcus (the nemesis of "strep throat" infections). Many of these strains are "hemolytic" meaning they cause microscopic bleeding in the gut. This can lead to fatigue due to undetected anemia. Sadly I see patients left untreated for these dysbiotic strains when they appear in their microbiology stool test results. Remember, their presence contributes to gut dysbiosis (the overgrowth of non-beneficial gut flora), leaky gut and chronic systemic inflammation.

Unless the doctor has found effective non-drug therapies, successful eradication of these chronic bacterial infections will not be possible. Unfortunately, in a majority of cases for my patients at least, those allopathic doctors shown lab results to verify the presence of streptococcus living in their colons responded to their patients by telling them these strains posed no threat. It was "ok" to have them there in their opinion! I can only suspect such a statement was made to the patient because allopathic medicine cannot eradicate these dysbiotic flora due to their drug resistance. As a result, they throw up their hands and tell the patient not to worry.

Every patient at Immune Matrix has a microbiology stool test done to identify dysbiotic strains. Every patient's dysbiotic strains are eradicated as part of their treatment protocol. Patients report that their child's behavior and focus significantly improves as well as their bowel movements once their streptococcus dysbiosis is eradicated. I have had patients resolve chronic headache and migraine. They report significant improvement in mental focus and clarity as well as improved digestive and joint function. They report experiencing less bloating, constipation and/or loose stools.

Re-inoculation is possible especially when the entire family has not been checked or treated. It can also occur due to food poisoning, or simply eating food contaminated from those who do not wash their hands after using the bathroom and then preparing food. When re-inoculation does occur, the patient is put back on a program of eradication. A blind eye is never turned to dysbiotic/pathogenic bacteria no more than you would knowingly leave a small cluster of termites in a foundation.

Eating one type of food daily and regularly often allows for that food to appear undigested in your blood stream when you have an overgrowth of dysbiotic flora creating leaky gut. Eating one food too frequently makes it easier for your immune system to recognize that food as "foreign". An inflammatory reaction to that food will then develop which can be so mild as to be unnoticeable unless one pays close attention to your energy level after eating the food. Remember too what I said about the immune system's reaction being spread thin over too many things to react to, making a reaction to any one thing diluted.

The greater the quantity and species of dysbiotic bacteria living in your digestive tract, the more "holes" it will have. The more likely you will develop digestive symptoms, food sensitivities and/or chronic fatigue and brain issues. How do you know if this is happening to you? One initial sign is feeling more tired an hour or two after eating. Other symptoms might include constipation, bloating, skin rashes, brain fog or irritability.

What if you take probiotics? Are you protected from these dysbiotic bacteria? Nope! Dysbiotic bacteria in the colon crowd out "good probiotics". It's like having weeds in a lawn! The more dysbiotic bacteria you have living in your colon, the more weeds in your lawn. You can throw the best grass seed onto that lawn. It won't take root because it's being crowed out by the weeds. The same goes for dysbiotic bacteria and good gut flora. Therefore, even if you are taking a probiotic, it cannot implant in your gut any more than throwing Kentucky Blue grass seed on a law full of weeds can thrive on a lawn full of weeds.

The more dysbiotic bacteria you have, the less good gut flora you will also have to make B12. With low B12 stores, you will have low energy and fatigue. Your liver will be unable to detoxify efficiently. It needs the B12 to process toxins. This also leads to fatigue as toxic overload hinders optimum organ and glandular function. Toxic retention slows metabolism, hinders biochemical reactions in the body and alters its acid/alkaline balance.

Does allopathic medicine test for the species and quantity of dysbiotic flora you have? No! Remember that allopathic medicine is focused on disease diagnosis. Dysbiosis is not a disease. It's a condition that could potentially lead to disease, but it is not considered a disease in and of itself. Allopathic medicine's focus is to identify "pathological infections". Unlike dysbiosis, most of the pathological infections of concern are acute and not chronic low grade or hidden infections.

For example, strep throat or helicobacter pylori (which causes ulcers) both act relatively quickly and severely initially. When the first course of antibiotics has quieted the infection such that it appears as if the entire infection is gone, some of the surviving pathogens set up house living in your digestive tract. Their growth over time can and does cause stomach pain, bloating, irritable bowel, constipation, loose stool, metabolic fatigue and food sensitivities.

The presence of these dysbiotic bacteria would not be detected but for the microbiology stool test I am referring to here. Furthermore, their elimination is not possible simply by taking another round of the same antibiotic. They have become drug resistant. Herbal/homeopathic remedies have proved to be the best resolve in what I have found in our clinics. These chronic infectious bacteria have set up house in your body to survive long term. They seek to evade detection to thrive. Thus, they are less likely to be detected by both the body and by traditional allopathic means.

In summary, you can easily stay stuck in your low energy trap due to allopathic oversight because it is less likely to eradicate chronic low grade bacterial infections for the following common reasons:

- allopathic medicine believes that the streptococcus pathogen is antibiotic resistant when found living in the gut and has no effective drug to eradicate these strains

- allopathic medicine believes that the streptococcus pathogen isn't causing harm when found living in the digestive tract! Many a doctor has told my patient that "It's no problem."

If you have a sore throat and go to the doctor, he/she will take a throat swab (hopefully!). When it is cultured, if they find streptococcus, you get a diagnosis of "strep throat". Sadly, more often than not, a patient is given an antibiotic without a culture. This is a key mechanism for how doctors create antibiotic resistant bacteria by trying to cut costs in running cultures. They then give prescriptions without doing a culture!

When you are given an antibiotic for "acute" strep throat infection, some bacteria will survive. While you had that glaring sore throat, your saliva contained these bacteria. You swallowed your saliva and inoculated your digestive tract with the streptococcus bacteria swimming in your saliva. Some of the streptococcus survived immune attack and set up house living in your colon. Some in time took up residence in your joints. Years later, those same strep throat bacteria can be living happily in your colon contributing to the formation of anemia, leaky gut, food sensitivities, and the progressive deterioration of your joints! Their continued presence leads to chronic low grade inflammation in your blood vessels contributing to plaque formation and hardening of the arteries. They can colonize on your heart valves and lead to inflexible heart valves, altering your cardiac output and effectiveness of valve closure. The bacterial colonies in your circulation and heart valves can dislodge and cause stroke and sudden death. If you survive, they leave you with long term disability. Depending upon where these bacteria set up house like termites, tissue degeneration and the gradual fatigue of your immune system will surely keep you in your low energy trap.

Your allopathic doctor will never think to look for the survival of those strep throat pathogens after having given you a course of antibiotics. The concept that they could even set up house in your colon evades most allopathic physicians. Even if another health care practitioner finds their presence with stool diagnostic testing, most allopathic doctors do nothing to eradicate it. I know this because my patients take the test results from our office to show their "other" doctor who says to them "oh, that's not a problem"! They ask me why their doctor didn't tell them the consequences of allowing these pathogens to thrive in their body, to my patients' dismay and my frustration. I hear this all the time. Yet once these same patients eradicate their dysbiosis they break through and out of many of their symptoms once and for all.

The circulation of the streptococcus family of pathogens among other dysbiotic flora is a significant cause for why so many people develop inflammatory disorders such as leaky gut, digestive disorders, arteriosclerosis, heart value inflammation and arthritis of the hip and fingers. When I would ask these doctors why nothing was done, they either tell me they "see it all the time", or they suspect or believe these strains are antibiotic resistant and know they have nothing they can prescribe the patient. Therefore, they tell the patient "it's no problem".

On several occasions we have seen doctors give their patients antibiotics in the hope of eradicating the gut streptococcus. It didn't make a dent in their level of gut streptococcus. We have seen through trial and error the difficulty in eradicating streptococcus from the digestive tract. While thirteen years ago it would take a month or two; it now can take several months to nearly a year! We at Immune Matrix have researched and tried various combinations of herbs, tinctures and homeopathics and can now assure all our patients that we have found a way to eradicate these strains from the gut despite their antibiotic resistance and persistence. In addition, we do everything we can to monitor sources of future infiltration.

Hidden bacterial infection has a significant impact upon fueling inflammation.

Immune Matrix has found chronic low grade bacterial infection to play a significant role with all patients suffering from inflammatory and immune driven conditions. Autism commonly involves various degrees of leaky gut and low grade brain inflammation, especially with recurrent ear infections. Headaches, migraine, developmental disorders involving auditory and verbal processing in children, and digestive issues involving food sensitivities can all find a common base of chronic low grade gut dysbiosis. Chronic low grade bacterial infection needs to be identified and rooted out if chronic inflammatory and immune driven disorders have any hope of sustained relief.

The best way to determine the "state" of your gut and whether low grade bacterial infection is contributing to inflammation and fatigue is to order a "microbiology stool" test by Doctor's Data. We at Immune Matrix consider this your "gut report card". The cost is very reasonable, under $100 as of this writing. You can order this test online through Immune Matrix's website at: https://www.immunematrix.com/store

This efficient and economical test is done in your home. You mail the sample directly to the lab. Within two weeks you get a "gut" report card showing the amount and types of strains of good probiotic flora living in your colon, as well as the pathogenic strains of bacteria, yeast, and candida. Furthermore, Doctor's Data cultures your pathogenic strains against prescription and non-prescription products to determine the best products needed to kill your strains, eliminating the guesswork so common in many clinical practices. The more pathogenic strains found and the greater the quantity of those strains, the more likely much of your inflammatory issues arise from leaky gut, which also leads to the development of hidden food sensitivities.

DiagnosTechs, a lab based in Kent Washington also runs GI panels with a library of over four thousand bacteria and fungi via state of the art MALDI-TOF apparatus used in only 5% of the labs in the United States. They use comprehensive markers for intestinal inflammation, including the presence of immunoglobulin antibodies to foods and parasites to hone in on the specific GI irritants. For more information go to their website at www.diagnostechs.com.

Other bacterial strains that keep you in your low energy trap are those associated with Lyme disease and their so-called co-infectants. These silent culprits of fatigue contribute to the development of chronic and serious degenerative symptoms and pathologies. Approximately 300 strains (and growing!) of organisms associate themselves with the "classic" Lyme pathogens of Borrelia, Babesia, and Ehrlichia.

Bartonella is found in cats and is transmitted to humans via their fleas. It is also transmitted to humans from mosquito and spider bites as well. I have found Bartonella to be the most resistant and persistent co-infectant associated with Lyme disease in my clinical experience. Anyone owning a cat, indoor or outdoor/indoor, should have it checked for Bartonella by their vet. It is the most difficult co-infectant to control, and total eradication is nearly impossible.

The entire Lyme disease family along with its co-infectants create a myriad of symptoms which span the gamut of joint pain, brain fog, malabsorption due to digestive disorders, heart arrhythmias, thyroid disorders, and fatigue, to name a few. Take a look at the symptom chart produced by Spiro Stat, a unique lab that tests for vector borne pathogens. By first selectively targeting parts of the genetic code of these organisms specific to unwanted bacteria found in your bodily fluids or tissue samples, this lab identifies a host of spirochete, bacterial and fungal pathogens.

Spiro Stat created this chart of symptoms we reproduced below.

Symptoms	Brachyspira	Coxiella	Spirillum	Babesia	Anaplasma	Afipia	Bartonella	Rickettsia	Ehrlichia	Ureaplasma	Francisella tularensis	mycoplasma	Leptospira	Treponema	Borrelia
Chemical Sensitivities															x
Muscle Twitching														x	x
Neuropathies														x	x
Paralysis														x	x
Numbness														x	x
Bone pain						x	x							x	x
Jaw pain						x	x							x	x
Hemorrhages	x				x				x		x				

Continual Infections						x	x							x	x
Uncontrollable Emotions												x	x	x	x
ADD								x		x			x	x	x
Drowsiness	x			x						x		x	x	x	x
Joint pain			x		x	x	x			x	x			x	x
Respiratory Problems		x		x	x				x	x	x	x	x		
Memory loss	x							x	x	x		x	x	x	x
Renal pain or Failure			x	x	x			x	x	x			x	x	x
Vision Eye issues						x	x	x	x		x	x	x	x	x
Swollen glands	x		x			x	x	x			x	x		x	x
Light sensitivity						x	x	x	x		x	x	x	x	x
Skin rashes			x		x	x	x	x	x		x		x	x	x
Fatigue	x	x	x	x				x		x	x	x	x	x	x
Disorientation Confusion	x	x		x	x			x	x	x		x	x	x	x
Nausea	x	x	x	x	x			x	x	x	x	x			x
Rigors chills		x	x	x	x	x	x	x	x	x	x	x			x
Abdominal pain	x	x		x	x	x	x	x	x	x	x	x			x
Headaches		x	x	x	x	x	x	x	x	x	x	x	x	x	x
Muscle pain		x	x	x	x	x	x	x	x	x	x	x	x	x	x
Malaise	x	x	x	x	x	x	x	x	x	x	x	x	x	x	x
fever	x	x	x	x	x	x	x	x	x	x	x	x	x	x	x

As you can see, you cannot determine which species of pathogen is causing your symptoms or their levels in your body. Many species of pathogens contribute to the same symptoms. To assume your problem is due to only one Lyme pathogen is to toss a dice and use that as your clinical assessment or try to be psychic! Many Lyme pathogens mimic the same symptoms.

Many non-lyme related pathogens also share the same symptoms! Many mold, bacterial and viral pathogens are confused for Lyme symptoms. Even more significant and tricky are the presence of fungal pathogens that mimic Lyme symptoms! Many a symptom is blamed on a Lyme pathogen when its culprit is dysbiotic fungal overgrowth in the body, often in the digestive tract. Symptoms such as brain fog, obsessive and dark thoughts, irritability and brain fatigue are also the legion of fungus and candida and not the sole dominion of Lyme pathogens.

Symptom alone cannot determine the identity of your pathogen species.

I cannot stress enough that you and your Lyme disease specialist are not psychic enough to determine which pathogen is causing your symptoms by description alone. Yet daily, assumptions are made by "Lyme specialists" who do not bother to order functional labs to identify pathogenic strains of bacteria, yeast, or fungus after the initial diagnosis of Lyme disease. Nor do they track viral titers of fatigue causing agents. They only focus on assuming the problem is principally due to Lyme pathogens and do not look to eliminate other contributing pathogens. Even those specialists that do appropriate lab work do so only for initial diagnosis and not to monitor effectiveness of their treatment protocol. Sadly, our laboratories only test for a handful of what truly comprises hundreds of strains! Do not let yourself be a victim of Lyme myopia. Good lab work is essential to monitor one's progress and eliminate all sources of pathogens that could keep you in your low energy trap.

Neither can you determine by symptom relief alone whether all the pathogens are gone, or that a specific strain has been eliminated. Sadly this is exactly the standard of care given in modern clinical medicine and among many specialists in the treatment of Lyme disease today. Why? This is most likely due to lack of better assessment parameters aside from relying upon symptoms alone. However, to base one's prescription and assessment of how well pathogens are being killed on symptom assessment alone is to play guesswork and roulette with which pathogen might be causing the actual problem. Is it no wonder pathogens slip through undetected and untreated and patients are overmedicated with multiple drug combinations and for extended periods of time?

Knowing which pathogens are causing which symptoms versus which symptoms arise due to the side-effects of treatments, toxic retention, or reactions to die off is essential. For example, Immune Matrix commonly finds overgrowth of yeast and candida contributing to the development of intestinal dysbiosis that leads to fatigue, lack of appetite, brain fog, brain fatigue as well as digestive symptoms. These same symptoms are often attributed to Lyme disease symptoms for which potent, costly and toxic prescription medications are prescribed for long term use.

Long term use of antibiotics is a substantial cause for yeast/candida/fungal overgrowth in the colon. However, too often Lyme pathogens are blamed for the continuing symptoms and the deteriorating digestive systems of those believed to be suffering from chronic Lyme disease. I commonly see Lyme patients put on antibiotics for 2 years or longer. No monitoring of their gut flora and no recommendation is given they take probiotics!

Lyme pathogens and their co-infectants can remain dormant and even morph (change) to a more virulent state, only to activate years later. They can cause even more severe symptoms than when originally contracted. It was only discovered a few years ago that Lyme pathogens can change their form and in doing so they became more drug resistant and therefore "virulent". It was surmised by some medical Lyme specialists that the antibiotics killed off the least resistant strains, stimulating the remaining pathogens to change structure to avoid detection. Of those pathogens that are not killed, the survivors become more virulent by nature of having been stimulated to survive by "morphing". This makes their detection and treatment in the long run more difficult. This is why working with Lyme-literate, experienced, and up to date experts who regularly treat the disorder and attend national conferences for the latest research developments is your best hope to manage this type of chronic infection. This is where to start.

However, human nature being what it is, specialists tend to see things through the lens of their specialty. As a result, a common oversight on the part of many such experts is to see everything through "Lyme" glasses and blame all symptoms on those pathogens. Little focus is placed on monitoring of gut pathogens and improving digestion. The result, hidden infection, in the form of gut dysbiosis, goes undetected. This in turn leads to the erosion of immune function, decreased glandular function, increased food and environmental sensitivities, brain neurotransmitter imbalances, increased toxic retention as well as increased reactivity to die-off of mycotoxins, molds, candida and bacteria. Any one of these is commonly mistaken for Lyme disease symptoms. It's not to say that Lyme pathogens will not affect these functions, however, independent and divergent metabolic imbalances play a significant role in manifesting these symptoms. Therefore, let us not leave one stone unturned.

Regular BIA monitoring will track your tissue regeneration progress.

Toxic retention from chronic harsh antibiotic treatment, accompanied with accelerated oxidative damage to tissue leads to accelerated tissue degeneration. Was the tissue degeneration caused by the pathogen or by chronic toxic retention and oxidative damage from microbial metabolites and/or long term harsh prescription drugs? With regular BIA monitoring one can catch this degenerative process early. I regularly observe the jump to assumption by doctors that their patients' Lyme disease is getting worse. In fact what has been occurring is one of two things. Other non-Lyme disease infections have gone undetected or the patient has not been able to regenerate and repair tissue in concert with the constant focus on anti-microbial protocols to the neglect of cellular nutrition and repair.

Uprooting the sources for low grade chronic bacterial infection will relieve the systemic burden they play in fatiguing not only the immune system but organ and glandular function as well. Like uprooting the weeds in one's lawn, eliminating all sources for bacterial infection will help ensure that bacteria are not a significant cause for keeping you in your low energy trap!

PART 6 – ATP AND YOUR MITOCHONDRIA

If you think of the furnace in your house as specialized machinery that keeps your home warm, the mitochondria are specialized living structures in your cells making the energy molecule known as ATP, adenosine-tri-phosphate. In the late 1950's Philip Siekevitz recognized this cell structure as the "powerhouse" of the cell. Mitochondria perform other key metabolic functions. For purposes of this book, our main 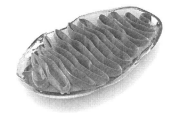 focus will be the energy molecule ATP. Mitochondria are the only cell structures that make ATP. Without ATP we cannot live, for it is the molecule of energy every cell in our body relies upon to thrive. The very food we eat is used in part for the eventual synthesis of this energy giving molecule that nourishes our cells.

The biochemical process by which this energy molecule ATP is made is very well mapped out. The molecular components of ATP synthesis is akin to a conveyor belt of molecules which include the need for key enzymes and ever increasing larger molecules (metabolites). Some of these metabolites cost the body more energy to make (expensive ingredients from an energy standpoint) and thus cost the body a certain amount of energy expenditure for the synthesis of essential components/ingredients for ATP synthesis. That ribbon you see inside the photograph of the mitochrondria functions like a conveyor belt to make ATP.

There is truly no other cell substitute for what our mitochondria do. So what could possibly go wrong here to keep us in our low energy trap? A few things can and do go wrong. First of all, if you struggle with your digestion to break down protein, carbohydrate and fat into simple amino acids, simple sugars and fatty acids, then your body will be lacking some core building blocks necessary for the citric acid aka Kreb's cycle whereby ATP is made in your mitochondria. This slows the production of energy your cells will have access to, necessary to their function. Fatigue and slow metabolic function anywhere in the body can result.

The first course of action given most patients whose astute doctors suspect a Kreb's cycle issue is to have them take B vitamins, possibly NADH too since this is one of the largest molecules at the end of the conveyor belt that converted to ATP. Giving NADH as a supplement saves the body the necessity of having to make NADH, a high energy and taxing molecule to synthesize. However, though many patients will feel a boost of energy and feel hope that this springs them out of their low energy trap, many for reasons described below, will find reducing returns the longer they stay on these products.

This leads us to the second issue I see with patients struggling from fatigue. Their immune system has become "sensitized" to some of the metabolites in the ATP synthesis cycle. Besides developing immune sensitivities to what you do not digest and break down well (proteins, sugars, fats, vitamins, minerals), you can develop immune sensitivities to any metabolite in any metabolic cycle, but more commonly to larger molecules such as NADH, ADP, and core metabolites that are essential to the process of making ATP.

How would you know if you are developing or already have an immune sensitivity to an ATP metabolite or ATP itself? There are certain supplements that can be given by doctors in the know to fill in the gaps to help someone synthesize more ATP and thus gain more energy. They include but are not limited to:

Amino acid supplementation
Fatty acid supplementation
NADH supplements
B vitamin/B12 supplementation
Oxaloacetate supplementation

You might initially feel better on these supplements but with leaky gut and hidden inflammation, over time your immune system can become "sensitized" to the supplement. This causes your body to react as if it were experiencing an allergy. Symptoms from rashes, headache, digestive upset, acid reflux, nausea, bloating, fatigue, brain fog to generalized malaise can result once your immune system has become sensitized to the supplement. Identifying a specific symptom can also be hard to do when you remember the example I gave you previously of macrophages that never get a chance to excrete enough histamine because they react to so many things thus diluting your immune reaction and masking your symptoms.

Your immune system can also become sensitized to an ingredient of the supplement. This results from inefficient break down/digestion of that supplement. You will then begin to feel worse on the supplement, a telltale sign of a possible immune sensitivity developing.

It is common for our clinics to find immune sensitivities develop to the B vitamins, the folate, the precursor molecules in the ATP synthesis cycle such as ADP, or NADPH. These sensitivities often arise more frequently in those individuals with genetic SNPs, defects per se. These SNPs make processing of the metabolite slower, giving the immune system a greater opportunity to "recognize" the metabolite as "foreign". This in turn makes digestion and absorption of that nutrient even more problematic. Ingesting that product will then turn on inflammatory reactions to that metabolite by nature of programmed immune recognition.

I know this has occurred in many of our patients with chronic and cyclical fatigue because we have developed a method to test the body for "sensitivity" to the key metabolites of the Kreb's cycle. We treat these sensitivities the way we would treat for food sensitivities. When we shut off the immune system's reactivity to the metabolite, the patient is then able to take the supplement and regain function in their ATP synthesis without side effects.

The third thing that could be happening is you have developed "mitochondrial disease", aka sick mitochondria. Unfortunately, the patients I have seen with this diagnosis were advised by their doctors this was a condition they would be stuck with. Before you go and tattoo this disease name to your arm please be aware the number of mitochondrial experts in the world are few and far between. You might be able to count them on your left hand. The few patients that receive any type of lab work for mitochondrial function get them through labs in Europe. Therefore, understand that testing is not readily accessible in this country nor do most health care practitioners have any knowledge about what makes mitochondria sick and how to test for and treat a patient with the myriad of problems that can arise with the Kreb's cycle.

Bear in mind also that the causes for "sick" mitochondria are multiple. Some individuals have genetic mutations that directly affect their mitochondria. When this occurs the problem often begins in childhood. Even with genetic mutations affecting mitochondrial function, bear in mind what you eat coupled with your environment can and does alter gene expression. Therefore, the body is capable of improving its function if you heed your diet, supplementation and toxic exposure.

Other individuals develop sick mitochondria over time as a result of infection. Viral infections seem to have the greatest impact according to my clinical observations. Chronic fatigue viruses such as Epstein Barr, cytomegalovirus, and echo virus can alter mitochondrial function. Lyme disease, co-infectants of Lyme, Rocky Mountain Spotted Fever and any pathogen that causes systemic infection, including insidious parasite-like organisms such as giardia and blastocystis, stachybotrys/aka black mold, chronic candida as well as fungal infections, all impact our mitochondria. All these pathogens can alter mitochondrial DNA.

Toxic retention can alter gene function, especially mitochondrial genes. Undigested food, pathogen die-off, by-products of drugs, supplements and environmental contaminants all contribute to toxic retention and free radical accumulation in the body. Free radicals are known to alter DNA structure and thus alter mitochondrial function.

The emerging science of what foods our red blood cells are unable to process and thus result in increasing one's toxic retention and gene alteration is significant and largely unrecognized in allopathic medicine. Dr. D'Adamo's latest research on red blood cells is hitting upon an important finding in the clue to why certain foods make certain individuals more toxic! His work in "genotyping" people beyond the study of eating for your blood type of A, AB, O, B and determining which foods for which genotype make that person retain toxic byproducts is probably the best groundbreaking research to enable each of us to minimize our toxic exposure and retention. What we eat daily is food or poison, nourishes and heals or adds to the daily dose of toxic retention that will cause/fuel our developing cancers and inflammatory conditions. His contribution in helping each of us to navigate away from foods that increase our toxic retention is hugely significant.

A simple change in diet can turn back the hands of time!

Since incorporating Dr. D'Adamo's work into our nutritional practice we have found remarkable changes in our patients' ability to ward off toxic retention and thus inflammation. Furthermore, avoiding those foods that make your genotype toxic can help to spring many a patient from their low energy trap. A simple change in the diet to avoid chicken if that is a "toxic" food for your genotype can turn back the hands of time in regaining youthful energy! I see it happen to our patients all the time!

Besides the viral, fungal, and free radical avenues our mitochondrial DNA can suffer damage from, there is also the emerging science of the genetic impact of our food in altering our genes. A prime example announced at one of the American Academy of Anti-Aging Medicine's conferences (A4M) was the study of eating gluten and its effect upon the brain. It was thought that eating wheat/gluten based products took approximately three weeks to exit the body. SPECT scans performed on brains showed that it took 6 months from one dose to clear the brain. These individuals did not test positive for celiac disease and yet manifested inflammatory changes in the brain that were detected to linger in the brain for six months! The entire auditorium, over two hundred doctors were told "If you value your brain, at least for the sake of your patients, go gluten free!" The groan in the audience was notable and this is from doctors who know better!

Another study published in Neurologic & Psychiatric Manifestations of Celiac Disease & Gluten Sensitivity also confirmed the six month time frame for significant reversals of brain inflammation and psychiatric symptoms in celiac patients! (Psychiatr Q. 2012 March; 83(1):91-102)

Therefore, if you or someone you know has avoided gluten for a month and not seen a difference in symptoms, consider this new information and extend the avoidance to six months.

More and more research is confirming the genetic link certain foods play in causing inflammation and gene alteration. Several proteins identified in wheat products besides gluten and gliadin are emerging culprits in creating the gene alterations we experience when we eat that food. In fact, the A4M conference I spoke of above illuminated the need for anyone to avoid gluten to reduce inflammation that could affect the brain. This is why any doctor telling you that you can eat gluten if you do not test positive for celiac is incorrect and out of date.

The International Celiac Disease Symposium in Oslo in 2011 officially differentiated Celiac Disease from Gluten Sensitivity. DiagnosTechs currently offers a GI-02 Health Panel to identify SIgA antigliadin antibodies with positive inflammatory markers linked to Celiac disease and distinguishes those from elevated inflammatory markers suggestive of only gluten sensitivity. However, glutenin is another gluten associated protein that is known to also trigger at least nine different genes in the body linked to chronic inflammation from infertility, skin disorders to brain fog. With ongoing research the long term health risks from the daily intake of gluten containing foods well warrants the expansion of gluten free food.

SPECT scans of the brain are confirming the inflammatory link and duration of time it takes to heal from eating high inflammatory food. Thus the food-gene connection to our gene alteration and its fueling our development of autoimmune disease, brain inflammation, and mitochondrial dysfunction cannot be ignored. This is why what we eat is so important and why our clinics at Immune Matrix make it an essential part of every patient's education to identify their toxic/inflammatory food triggers to help them reduce all sources for inflammation and toxic retention.

In summary, a significant element of *Escaping Your Low Energy Trap* is to improve ATP synthesis and usage. Know what supplements benefit ATP/mitochondrial function. Determine if you have internal metabolic resistances to taking such supplements that could suggest your immune system has become reactive to key metabolites. If so, get treated. Lastly, identify hidden sources for infection. Just as termites erode a home, infection will surely derail your mitochondrial function over time.

PART 7 – MOLD SENSITIVITIES

Mold has various effects upon the body. When I speak of mold, I'm speaking in broad terms to include yeast, candida, fungal exposures and overgrowths. There are food related "molds" that associate with the plant as it grows and matures. Examples are smut and bunt molds, found in corn, oats and wheat. They cannot be washed off the food! Many

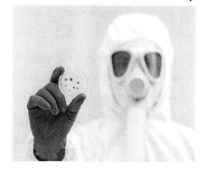

individuals react to the smut or bunt in these food products as opposed to the sugar as in corn sugar, or protein, as in oat proteins. Other foods that contain high concentrations of mold by their very nature are grapes, cantaloupe, honeydew melon, raisins, and strawberries. We refer to these foods at Immune Matrix clinics as the "moldy foods". We advise anyone suffering from food sensitivities, chronic inflammation, allergies, autism, asthma, eczema, irritable bowel, Lyme disease and/or brain fog to especially steer clear of these otherwise tasty "moldy" foods.

Mold sensitivities are immune sensitivities that cause allergy-like symptoms. Symptoms include but are not limited to brain fog, sleepiness, rage or aggressive behavior after exposure to food or environmental borne molds, sugar cravings, insomnia, racing thoughts, skin rashes, bloating and fatigue.

Besides the molds in food discussed above, mold in your home (bathroom mold from sinks and showers), hidden black mold (stachybotrys), pathogenic molds that live in your body such as Candida, indoor/outdoor molds that live in soil (aspergillas – also found in cigarette smoke), and those that live in fallen tree leaves/compost, can all trigger immune sensitivities. Mold sensitivities will then trigger inflammation anywhere in the body and sap your immune system and body of vital energy.

Molds, fungus and yeast can have an intense acute effect upon the body. These cases are easy to identify and treat. Thrush and vaginal yeast are common examples. However, just with chronic viral and bacterial infections, molds, fungus and yeast can have very subtle very chronic effects upon the body. These cases are largely missed and their significance is underappreciated by most allopathic doctors. However, identifying reactivity to mycotoxins, molds, yeast and/or candida could be essential to whether you recover from your low energy trap.

If the presence of pathogenic fungus inside your body were not enough, mycotoxins, their excretions, are another huge immune sensitizing issue. Some mycotoxins are natural excretions from the byproducts of metabolism of these creatures. Other mycotoxins result from their death, die-off that needs to be excreted by the body or it becomes retained in tissues. Mycotoxins are also used in the food industry to give some cheese their distinctive flavor! Roquefort cheese is such an example.

Mycotoxins are inflammatory to the brains of mold sensitive individuals. They cause neurological issues. Sudden brain fog, hyperactivity, fatigue, sudden anger and aggressive behavior, irritability, restlessness, insomnia, racing thoughts, headache, and malaise are a few examples of mold sensitivity symptoms. Don't they also sound like food sensitivity, multiple chemical sensitivity and Lyme disease symptoms? The common thread is they all trigger immune reactions and these reactions can affect many of the same areas of the body.

Mycotoxin sensitivity is a primary reason why many a patient is unable to eradicate mold/candida pathogens from their body. Here is a brief list of common mycotoxins: butenolide, trichodermin, trichoverrins, emodin, cytochalasin E, vomitoxin, destruxin B, trochoverrols, verruculogen, viomellein, slaframine, citreoviridin, alternariol methyl ether, cyclosporin A, penicillic acid, ochratoxin, fusric acid, tunuazonic acid, trichothecin, neosolaniol, acetaldehyde, fusarin, diacetoxyscirpenol, xanthocillin, zearalenone, cephalosphorin C, cyclopiazonic acid, roquefortine C, fumagilin, nivalenol, islanditoxin, HT-2 toxin, sterigmatocystin, alternariol, cotocin, penitrem A, lycomarasmin, fumonisin viriditoxin, kojic acid, ipomeanine, aflatoxin, rubatoxin, lateirin, amanitins, malformin, penicillin, verucanns, cochliodinol, patulin, satratoxins, austdiol, gliotoxin, T2 toxin, austamide, citrinin, brevianamide, roridin E, moniliformin, griseofulvin, avenacein, monoacetoxyscirpenol, rugulosin, ergot, acetyldeoxynivalenol, aflatrem, beauvericin, oxalic acid, chatoglobosin, and calonectrin.

Too aggressive a treatment protocol for candida/fungus/Lyme disease treatment can cause an elevation of these mycotoxins in the body from die-off of pathogens. What is too aggressive a treatment? I generally say when you start to feel worse the longer you are on a program. The underlying problem often is that you're not excreting the byproducts of die-off and medications and therefore your toxic retention is increasing. Aggravation of symptoms can result. This often leads the patient to stop the treatment as they become more reactive with time. Mycotoxins are thus another fundamental and little recognized cause for chronic fatigue in those individuals that cannot excrete/detoxify from the die-off of mold/yeast/candida.

Many a patient copes with their reactivity to die-off and mold/candida exposure by taking activated charcoal, PectaSol, and even prescription cholestyramine to help soak up the mycotoxins. Others use coffee enemas to help their liver cope with detoxification. However, when the reactivity is severe, many a patient has to stop treatment or significantly slow their pathogen eradication program in order to control the side-effects of toxic retention. Some give up entirely. Those are the patients I most often see.

Furthermore, patients with the most severe immune sensitivities to molds and mycotoxins tend to have the most severe reactions. These patients have livers congested and stressed with microbial metabolites. Their immune reactivity to mycotoxins is severe with the least amount of die-off. Our Immune Matrix clinics de-sensitizes patients to mycotoxin sensitivities as well to the pathogen(s) they tested "sensitive" to, while simultaneously improving and eliminating their toxic retention. This seems to help those patients who could not previously handle molds/

candida and mycotoxin die-off. They are then capable of embarking and following through on an effective treatment program. The patients were able to take anti-fungal prescription and non-prescription formulas for the first time in years to overcome their chronic low grade infections and do so for a shorter period of time to finally escape their low energy trap. As a result, they emerged from their other symptoms with a new state of health.

8 – TOXIC RETENTION

The subject of how toxins affect the body, which type of toxins cause us the most trouble, our biochemical challenges in excreting these toxins, how and where the body retains toxins and their long term effects upon health are all a relatively new and emerging science. The greatest inroads in these areas have come through the field of functional and alternative medicine through those practitioners that treat autism and Lyme disease and those that help patients detoxify heavy metals aka chelation doctors. I am excited about the continuing evolution and development of this field. It is proving to have a significant impact in altering the course of chronic inflammatory conditions. I have seen it help many a patient to overcome chronic infection and escape their low energy trap!

Toxic retention is a huge source of fatigue that is not routinely addressed as part of one's health care program in most medical systems. Yet toxins retained in the body can reduce the vitality of our tissue and organ function and impede nutrient absorption. Without optimal nutrient absorption on a cellular level, and without optimal organ and glandular function, you will surely stay in your low energy trap!

Toxins have various sources. The air we breathe contains contaminants from industrial off gassing as well as the byproducts from the fuel we use to power our cars. Lead in leaded gasoline for our cars are a prime source for daily lead exposure. Over time, the toxic retention of lead will lead to arteriosclerosis and hypertension among other chronic debilitating health conditions.

After Japan's nuclear plant melt down, I also started to see increases in radiation exposure, especially uranium markers here in California. I immediately began to monitor as many of my patients as I could, myself included. For several months the radiation markers I was following made a steady climb upward. Though the levels were well below the published limit for safety, no amount of constant radiation exposure is without risk. It was a cause for concern whether our bodies would be capable of keeping up with the increased radiation exposure, even with detoxification agents. Luckily, with quick trial and error I did find an effective solution to reducing the toxic retention of radiation in myself and my patients.

Besides circulating in the air we breathe, toxins are found as contaminants in the food we eat. Every pesticide, herbicide, industrial pollutant that rains down upon our crops, the chemical fertilizers used on organic and non-organic crops to boost our depleted soil nutrients all make their way into our bodies. These food contaminants need to be excreted by our body or stored for safe keeping. Certainly eating organic significantly reduces the contaminant load (and greatly increases the nutrient load). However, how the food is prepared is equally significant in determining whether a fungicide sprayed by customs on an imported spice used by a restaurant becomes a toxin that is unknowingly and silently added to our bodies. Fungicides, pesticides, herbicides, food additives, food preservatives, stabilizers, flavor enhancers and colorings all exact a toxic toll on how much toxic retention we can handle and excrete.

In the process of educating our patients to eliminate processed foods from their diets, many found their hypertension disappearing and their weight melting off without additional effort. Conditions besides fatigue, such as those involving food sensitivities, rashes and digestive issues resolve when the immune trigger, the food "contaminant" is eliminated from the diet.

An interesting example was a child we treated who had a favorite pizza restaurant. He would regularly suffer a nose bleed after eating their pizza. Her mother brought the child to me for food sensitivity testing and we discovered a particular food preservative used in the cheese.

Toxins also enter our body through the environment. Industrial pollution, synthetic perfumes, flame retardants put into the fabric of our clothing, bedding, and furnishings provide daily exposure to young and old alike. We breathe, touch or ingest these toxins. The off-gassing of chemicals from paint solvents, pressed wood use to manufacture housing, refrigeration, gas stoves, carpet off gas, plastic products, glues and fixatives used in flooring to the chemicals in our laundry, soap, cosmetics, skin care, hair dyes, furnace and fireplace fumes and cleaning detergents all add to our toxic retention. Don't forget the petrochemicals and BHA contaminants in the plastic water bottles we drink from.

Toxins also come from the byproducts of our digestion. This can occur because we lack sufficient enzymes and/or stomach acid to break down protein, carbohydrate and/or fats into simple amino acids, simple sugars and simple fatty acids. Other products of digestion will also lead to our developing food sensitivities when they are not broken down into their simple components. This is how we develop food sensitivities, from the foods we eat most frequently when we do not digest them well. Our lack of digestive ability for food and those additives and associated chemicals, where the breakdown is not complete and sufficient to allow the body to absorb it on a cellular level, then becomes part of the toxic sludge we either retain or excrete. Undigested and improperly digested food therefore adds to our daily toxic load.

Some of us have more problems breaking down toxins and excreting them. Dr. D'Adamo recently coined the term "secretor" and "non-secretor" to refer to the red blood cell's ability to secrete its blood type antigen. The significance of this finding is that "non-secretors" we have found, are slower detoxifiers, have more lymphatic congestion and process drugs and pill supplements slower than "secretors". For our work with toxic, chronically ill patients, this is a significant barometer.

We have found that non-secretors tend to be more severely ill, are more likely to suffer chronic infection, low glandular function, digestive issues, brain symptoms and low energy as well. They are also the patients that need the most hand-holding in order to get them out of their low energy trap. They are also the most likely to have side effects from a doctor's treatment protocol whether it's from drugs, vitamins, herbs or homeopathics!

*Non-secretors are the most challenged to
process medication, supplements & to detoxify.*

Finding out if you are a non-secretor is important. If you would like to order this kit, please contact us at one of our clinics or through our website (www.immunematrix.com online store – non-secretor test). The test is simple, done in your home and mailed out with your saliva sample. It takes approximately two weeks to obtain the results. Once you know if you are a secretor or non-secretor, there is no re-testing. You are a secretor or non-secretor for life.

Knowing that you need to have additional lymphatic drainage and detoxification support as a non-secretor will help you immensely to handle any antibiotic treatment protocol, prescription drug or supplement program any doctor may need to put you on. Your only problem will be finding a practitioner knowledgeable in drainage to assist you while you are on your treatment protocol.

Knowing if you are a non-secretor is also a red flag that your diet needs to focus on avoiding those foods that make you toxic! This information can be determined once you find out what your "genotype" is. Do not try to determine your genotype from reading Dr. D'Adamo's book alone as you will be tempted to go by symptoms alone. This is very misleading. Even I fell into that trap and was greatly surprised when my certified genotype nutritionist advised me after doing the calculations from my measurements and analyzing other parameters that my assumption was not even close when based on reading the book alone for its symptoms! What I thought I was from the descriptions of the genotypes turned out to be 100% wrong. Therefore, make no assumptions. Get tested and know the truth.

Knowing if you are a non-secretor and what genotype you are will help spring you out of your low energy trap. In my own case, just avoiding the foods toxic for my genotype helped me to lose weight I thought I'd never loose and surprisingly helped spring my energy back more than ten years! This alone could very well be your missing link to finally improving glandular function and metabolism.

Becoming aware of your digestive challenges will also help you minimize your toxic retention. Lack of digestive breakdown of otherwise clean and healthy food will also add to your toxic retention. For example, if you had your gallbladder removed, your ability to break down oils and fats is greatly hindered. Your body still needs fatty acids from fats/oils to repair tissue and regenerate nerve/brain tissue. However, your inability to break down these fats will cause you to retain these undigested fragments of digestion as toxins quicker than someone with an intact gallbladder. Therefore, toxins can come from good healthy food we eat when we are unable to digest it as well as from contaminants in our food and environment.

Toxins do not have to be ingested. Just as toxins can be breathed in from the air, they can also be absorbed through our skin. For example, there are chemicals in the paper that merchants print receipts on that become absorbed through our skin on contact. In that brief moment that you hold the receipt, your skin comes into contact with a chemical known as bisphenol A or BPA. Their effect is known to alter our fat metabolism, causing us to gain weight as well as adding to our toxic load among other hideous things. (http://link.springer.com/article/ 10.1007%2Fs00216-010-3936-9) This is also how we absorb flame retardant chemicals, through contact with skin in treated clothing and furnishings required by law on all baby and children fabric and household furnishings.

By and large, anything we don't excrete or have trouble excreting becomes a toxin. It then needs to be neutralized, excreted or stored by the body if it cannot be excreted. This includes the byproducts of what we eat: the over the counter medications and prescription medications, the vitamins and supplements, herbal remedies, the pathogens our body kills, and the preservatives and adjuvants (aluminum, thimerisol aka mercury) in our vaccines. Hormones in face creams (like progesterone because it plumps the skin, undisclosed and allowed by our government), hormones we are prescribed, chemicals in lotions, soaps, detergents, and dry cleaning solvents left in our clothing all make contact with our skin. All of this needs to be eliminated by our body!

Toxins can accumulate in any tissue in the body when not appropriately excreted through urine or stools. Toxins can affect the brain, digestive tract and alter hormone and other metabolic processes leading to fatigue. Toxins can trigger inflammatory disorders such as environmental sensitivities and allergies. These conditions cause a host of symptoms that include fatigue.

Toxins (especially heavy metals like mercury, methy mercury (in seafood) and sodium ethyl mercury (in vaccines) make us acidic, allowing for the chronic growth and overgrowth of pathogens in our body. Toxic retention provides the perfect acidic home for dysbiotic bacteria to thrive in our colon, for mycoplasma to set up house and linger for months to years in our lungs long after that upper respiratory infection has passed. Spirochetes transmitted from fleas, ticks, spiders and mosquito bites and sexual transmission can swim in our bodies for years largely undetected blooming when the acid environment is just right for them to flourish. The chronic fatigue family of viruses, cytomegalovirus, echo virus and Epstein Barr virus, along with fungus, yeast and candida, and Lyme disease and their associated co-infectants all eat away at our bodies like termites in the basement especially when we become toxic.

Finally toxins can cause low hormone production in the body leading to chronic or cyclical fatigue. Have you ever gone to an aquarium store and seen an aquarium where the filter was clogged and the water became cloudy? Did you notice that the fish were lethargic despite being fed top grade live brine shrimp? And did you notice that once the water was sparkling clean, the same fish perked up and zipped around with zest? That is how we react when toxic retention pollutes our blood and lymphatic fluid. Our circulation slows ever so slightly. Our tissues, glands and organs receive less oxygen in "thicker" blood/fluids. Our blood and lymphatic fluid ph become ever so slightly more acidic which inactivates the enzymes in our body that help us to use hormones. Therefore, in an acid environment, we may make enough hormones and our blood tests will show normal levels of hormones but because our circulation and tissues are more acidic, we lack sufficient amount of functional enzymes (their being inactivated by an acid environment) to allow our body to use the hormones. This fact will escape your doctor who is only looking at your blood test. Fatigue is one result when we cannot use our hormones or we don't make enough.

Hormone replacement therapy is another source for toxic retention as is synthetic vitamin supplementation. In both cases the body has to take this non-natural form of hormone/vitamin and break it down and convert it to a usable form. This conversion process involves metabolic debris. If your liver detoxification pathways have major or minor genetic roadblocks to the smooth and timely metabolic processing of toxins in general, then your body will be slower at excreting synthetic hormones and supplements. If you unknowingly do not supply your body with the additional metabolic nutritional factors to help the liver detoxify, then you can further frustrate your body's efforts to eliminate these toxins. All of this has to be factored into the equation in determining your metabolic efficiency in detoxification and its contribution to making you acidic, inhibiting your ability to use hormones, and interfering with metabolism of energy producing glands.

Take a look at the chart on the next page. It depicts our typical daily source of toxic exposure. Our liver works 24/7 to keep up with our daily exposure. As you can see toxins come at us from sources that didn't exist a generation ago!

There is a huge difference between "poisoning" from toxic exposure versus chronic low grade toxic retention. Chronic toxic retention is not given much attention or merit in allopathic disease systems, yet it is even more significant in its impact upon our long term health and its contribution to making us susceptible to chronic infections, low hormone function, and thus chronic low energy.

Traditionally allopathic medicine only takes notice when the level of toxic accumulation amounts to a "poisoning". Examples are arsenic and lead poisoning. Symptoms would be ascribed to the effects of having been "poisoned" by the toxin. Blood tests would verify elevated "circulating" levels of these toxins to confirm poisoning. However, in the case of slow and gradual toxic accumulation, elevated blood levels of these toxins are lacking because they have been stored in tissues! Symptoms too are different than those of acute poisoning even for the same "poison".

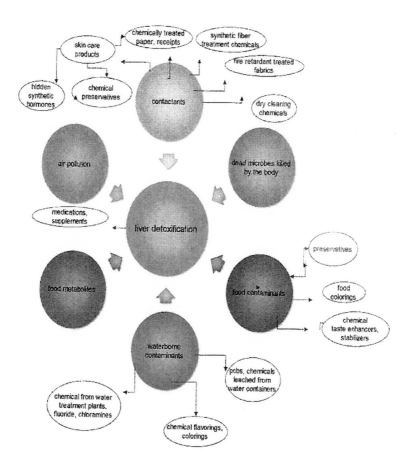

A classic example of "acute" poisoning is lead "poisoning". Acute lead poisoning paints a different symptomatic picture than that of slow toxic accumulation from lead. These acute cases are more common among children versus adults and the symptoms of acute lead "poisoning" are vastly different than chronic low grade toxic retention of lead. The toxic retention of lead that results from a slow and gradual accumulation over an extended period of time can amount to a "poisoning" eventually. However, this does not typically result in a "poisoning" due to the body's efficiency in storing and thus locking away the lead. The stored lead will have a significant impact on developing arteriosclerosis and bone disorders over time. Therefore, the fact the body stores the heavy metal is little consolation for its toxic effect.

Acknowledgement and recognition that symptoms from toxic retention commonly run silent is often neglected in the face of other more glaring and pressing "acute" symptoms in allopathic medicine. As a result, acknowledging and addressing the effects these hidden toxins have upon organ function and the role they play in developing other more chronic organ pathologies is not an allopathic focus unless it amounts to toxic "poisoning". Furthermore, when allopathic medicine's reaction to toxins is in the limited frame of toxic "poisoning" as in examples of arsenic or lead poisoning, it only looks for the specific and isolated symptoms associated with poisoning and not the subtle but equally baffling symptoms of slow toxic retention of those metals. Furthermore, allopathic medicine sees that one substance as one toxin causing xyz symptoms and not a myriad of toxins triggering and affecting entire metabolic and immune dysfunctions.

> *There is a huge difference between*
> *toxic poisoning and toxic retention.*

In the case of toxic retention, you have a multitude of toxins retained by the body whose cumulative effect can cause innumerable symptoms that can even mimic other disease states. For example, heavy metal retention in the brain can cause dementia-like symptoms: short term memory lapses, lack of focus and attention, brain fatigue, slurring of speech, headache and irritable mood swings and short tempers. Can you determine from these symptoms which heavy metal is the culprit, whether it is aluminum, mercury or some other heavy metal? Can you tell by symptoms alone that they are due to heavy metals and not in part or whole from mycotoxins, die-off of Lyme, fungal or bacterial pathogens? No. Not by symptoms alone.

The toxic retention of an overabundance of one metal such as lead or aluminum can cause the same symptoms as can the toxic retention of a general mix of heavy metals. Furthermore, short term memory loss, shorter attention spans, shifts in mood toward increased moodiness, agitation, shorter tempers, insomnia, anxiety and forgetfulness can all stem from toxic retention of heavy metals as much as they can also be caused by immune sensitivities to molds and mycotoxins or a simple deficiency of sex hormones, DHA and/or omega 3 fish oil!

Fear not however, there are ways to determine your heavy metal load and there are ways to safely eliminate a toxic burden. Chelation doctors specialize in heavy metal removal. However, those that are M.D.s are coming under attack more and more by the American Medical Association for practicing outside the disease paradigm. Doctors have to receive additional training to chelate patients, yet the AMA would rather have us wait until some disease strikes rather than reduce our risk by eliminating our toxic heavy metal burden while we safely and slowly can. Sadly, the AMA's intimidation of M.D.s is slowly working as I see more "chelation" doctors limiting their work or stopping the practice altogether.

Alternative and integrative specialists do exist with knowledge and experience to safely help you reduce your toxic retention. With appropriate follow up lab testing one can easily be monitored during the entire chelation process. In addition, with the advancement of supplement manufacturing processes, more options are now available to safely eliminate heavy metals with oral supplements with options to focus on stool excretion instead of urinary/kidney excretion pathways. It is now very safe through these modalities to chelate slowly and daily for adults as well as children.

Much has been investigated about the effects of aluminum on the brain as contributing to dementia-like symptoms. Does this mean the person has no other cause for their dementia? No, but it makes it difficult for medicine to use its "hole in the peg" methodology in diagnosing disease based on " x" as opposed to "y" when a multitude of toxins including lead and mercury in its various forms (methy, sodium ethyl and phenyl mercury) are "poisoning" and derailing your immune system function, fueling inflammation, increasing free radical development, all detrimentally affecting your metabolism albeit slowly! Therefore beware the doctor that tells you that you do not have an issue with heavy metals or other toxic retention when their view of toxicity encompasses only acute poisoning.

A toxin doesn't have to reach "poison" levels to have detrimental symptoms.

The prevalent allopathic view of **toxic poisoning** is one significant reason why testing for **toxic retention** is nearly impossible unless it becomes and amounts to a "poisoning". As a result, most allopathic physicians will not think to consider the impact of toxic retention in the evaluation of any medical condition yet alone a condition such as chronic fatigue or vague brain fog symptomatology where it often has a significant impact. Should they suspect some type of toxic exposure, they would be hard pressed to determine the type of exposure in order to determine the proper specialty lab to order a "poison" test.

A toxin doesn't have to reach "poison" levels tested in labs to have detrimental symptoms. In situations of acute toxic exposure, you will see circulating levels of that toxin in the blood stream and thus it can be found with blood testing. However, slower, low grade and chronic exposure to a toxin allows the body to store what it cannot excrete. Therefore that toxin will not show up in the same blood test that one sees for acute toxic poisoning. Does it mean you don't harbor significant levels of heavy metals that could derail your health? Obviously no, in fact toxins locked up in tissue cause the most damage.

Now I am sure you are beginning to understand why slow and gradual poisoning of our bodies from a myriad of toxins goes undetected and can keep us in our low energy trap! It also explains how one can have a clean blood lab result when testing for toxic metal poisoning and yet have tissues/glands/organs saturated with the heavy metal stocked away in the intracellular matrix (inside the cell), the intercellular matrix (in between the cells in the cellular matrix, what holds the cells connected to each other), or in the extra cellular matrix (the lymphatic fluid that moistens, nourishes and bathes our cells). Serum (blood) levels will simply not reflect intra/inter and extracellular toxic retention levels.

Aside from the food we eat and our inability to completely digest and use the food as a result, components of food digestion called metabolites become toxins for our bodies as do the pathogens (microbes) our body kills. Other metabolites form from the microbes we kill. Sometimes our body is not efficient at breaking down the microbes it kills and this hinders excretion. Both food and microbial metabolites have to be excreted or they will find a place to be retained and stored in the body. The colon and liver are common organs that retain larger metabolites. Any other tissue or organ can retain metabolites.

With respect to the toxic retention of mold metabolites and mycotoxins, their effect upon the body comes from their excretions (mycotoxins) and their overgrowth. Thus the inflammation they cause to tissue from their overgrowth and excretions is a byproduct of our body's inability to eliminate them and their excretions, aka toxic retention.

The more of these microbial metabolites you retain the more their chemical messengers can go to work in your body to alter metabolic function. For example, candida mycotoxins are chemical messengers that function to cause you to "feed" them by craving sweets! Even understanding that mold/candida pathogens cause certain symptoms, the distinction in understanding when symptoms are due to active infection versus our lack of excretion of their toxins from their die-off has had little recognition in medicine. It is as if it is presumed that we all excrete the byproducts of killing off pathogens and we all do it equally well. By now you know that this simply isn't true. The consequences of this oversight by medical practitioners is that many a patient is suspected to harbor symptoms from pathogens when the symptoms stem from an inability to excrete the byproducts of the die-off aka microbial metabolites.

How does one test for toxic retention of mold pathogens, other microbial metabolites and know what type to test for? How do you know what to suspect? Do you suspect the pathogen, their mycotoxin, a food metabolite sensitivity such as sulfur (that affects liver detoxification efficiency), heavy metals, and what type? There are many questions to ask. A seasoned practitioner experienced in distinguishing symptoms of detoxification pathway issues versus symptoms of toxic accumulation and their types versus symptoms caused by the metabolic effects of pathogens and their toxic retention may be crucial to your uncovering all sources for your fatigue.

Working with a practitioner who regularly tests for toxic exposure of different types and knows how to help the body safely excrete those toxins is your best recourse. Your body will be better able to bind and excrete specific toxins once you have identified the types of toxic stressors your body is under and you have been properly evaluated for your body's capacity and efficiency to bind and excrete the various toxins.

When can excretion of toxins become a problem? Excretion of toxins does not occur efficiently if your immune system has become "reactive" to some of the "toxins". Few medical practitioners understand the nuances of how the immune system can interfere with detoxification. I have spent the last thirteen years sharing my findings with doctors about the immune system's ability to shut down one's excretion of heavy metals. From that we have learned *the immune system can alter detoxification pathway/metabolic function.* Here are some questions to use as guidelines to go by in finding a practitioner to assist you in determining the nature and extent of your toxic burden:

1. What type of tests do they use to determine toxic accumulation
2. What type of toxins do they look for
3. Can they help your body be more efficient in detoxification, processing specific toxins?
4. Can they identify the specific nutrients your body needs to balance your methylation pathways
5. Can they identify where your immune system is interfering with methylation
6. Do they consider and are they educated in dealing with genetic SNPs (defects) affecting detoxification and do they know how to recognize the signs for such issues in patients, as well as know how to navigate around those issues?
7. What range of products do they use for the different toxins a person needs to excrete?
8. What labs do they use to monitor excretion types and amounts?

9. What do they do when a patient feels sicker while trying to detox on their protocol and how do they safeguard from such side effects

10. Does the practitioner practice a one style protocol for everyone?

If you would like more detailed information about detoxification and pathway information consult our blog: www.chronicfatigueandnutrition. com It offers information based upon the clinical experience of Immune Matrix's collective patient base over a dozen plus years with respect to toxins, toxicity, detoxification pathway issues and the effects toxicity and the immune system have in supporting and interfering with basic metabolic functions of the body. Articles are published regularly to provide you with the latest clinical outcomes and findings in the hope that this knowledge will empower you to find answers and improve the medical dialogue you have with your treating practitioner.

PART 9 – BRAIN CHEMISTRY

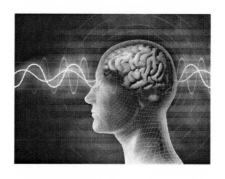

When I speak of brain chemistry, I'm talking about our neurotransmitters, the chemical signals that allow our brain cells to communicate with one another and the body. These chemical signals affect how we feel emotionally and mentally. They affect our ability to feel joy, modulate our ability to react to stress, our ability to become aroused and experience orgasms, to feel hungry or satisfied after a meal, to communicate our needs, wants and desires, and influence our creative expression. They determine how fast our brain processes visual and auditory information and our ability to maintain prolonged focus on task. They determine the rate in which we process nutrients and energy, burn fat, as well as the speed and quality of our thoughts. They regulate the duration and quality of our sleep, our perception of pain and pleasure, the nature and quality of our movement among thousands of other biological functions. These chemical signals also affect the body through a chemical communication network, communicating with glands to control our metabolism, modulating our heart rate, digestion and immune system function.

Brain chemistry and brain waves can either or both throw off the body's metabolic/immune balance.

Without properly balanced brain chemistry, imbalances in both the brain and body result. When certain aspects of our brain chemistry are out of balance, for example, when we don't make enough of a certain neurotransmitter, such as dopamine, we can become slow in movement and thought and our mood can become dark as if anticipating impending doom or a sense of "what does it matter". We can develop a dark mood for no reason, a feeling of doom and gloom that is chemically driven by the lack of sufficient amounts of dopamine and other neurotransmitters. This can also cause us to be tired, maybe even in a fatalistic "what's the use" sort of way that comes and goes with the ebb and flow of insufficient quantities of key neurotransmitters.

Sex hormones estrogen and testosterone also play into the workings of our brain chemistry. Low sex hormone production can take the very life and spark out of our brains besides the bedroom. Our brain and body become couch potatoes, feeling listless, unmotivated, and foggy at times. We might mistake these symptoms as signs of aging. Aging surely can aggravate those symptoms but not necessarily cause them. There may be a heaviness and fatigue that takes over for no apparent reason, even after having slept through the night. Women need access to estrogen for proper brain function. Men need access to testosterone. If there is an insufficient quantity of these hormones in the brain as opposed to the body, then brain and mood dysfunction or disorders can result. Sleep, focus, alertness, and vitality all decline.

Other neurotransmitters also affect our mood and therefore our energy. Low serotonin can make us feel blue, sad for no reason. We feel we've lost our joy in life even when we have every reason to be joyful.

Feeling sad and blue does depress our energy. It may simply be that nothing excites us like it used to, that we've lost our joy. Feeling sad and blue slows and congests the flow of energy called chi/qi that courses through every organ. It slows the energetic link to every organ/system in the body. In Chinese Medicine it is said that stagnation leads to disease much in the way that stagnant water in a pond leads to pollution and eventual decay and death of its inhabitants.

GABA, another neurotransmitter, when low, can make us feel edgy, even anxious, compounding fatigue while being edgy or wired. Low GABA is also responsible for panic disorders. Having adequate amounts of GABA, but not being able to use it well (because it is not well transported across our cell membranes), is another common problem that can lead to the same outcome but for a different mechanism. In addition, I commonly find many of my patients who suffer from inflammatory disorders/infections have developed an immune sensitivity to GABA which when reversed allows the patient to take supplements that increase its production and usage.

Elevated neurochemistry can also indirectly keep you locked in your low energy trap. Elevated stimulatory neurotransmitters such as dopamine, epinephrine, norepinephrine and glutamate can overstimulate you. It's as if you are parked in a garage, the car engine is on and your foot is on the brake and the gas. You may not be able to relax sufficiently to get to sleep as your engine is on and running fast, leaving you feeling wired and tired. The result is one's sleep cycle and quality of sleep will suffer. Excessive stimulatory neurotransmitters can also wear down your glandular function, leading to hypo-glandular, low hormone functions. Rebalancing the neurotransmitters will not necessarily result in glands popping back into normal function without additional treatment, but it will remove the suppressing function exhausting them.

As you can see, brain chemistry, when not balanced, leads to emotional and neurological symptoms. It can also affect the body and its functions. The challenge traditionally with allopathic medicine has been with its compartmentalization of organ and disease states. The body is viewed separate from the brain and treated that way also! We have the body doctors and the brain doctors, the neurologists, psychiatrists and psychologists. However, the two rarely coordinate efforts when a bodily condition affects the brain or when the brain detrimentally affects bodily functions. The result from this lack of integration of seeing the brain/body dynamics as a whole is to miss out on key opportunities to improve bodily function by optimizing brain chemistry and improve brain function/ disorders by optimizing body chemistry.

If you thought brain chemistry and its effect upon contributing to bodily disorders such as chronic fatigue, weight gain, heart and thyroid issues is complicated, consider the subject of brain wave frequency. Our brains send out different frequencies to correspond to different brain/body functions. Alpha waves at 9-13 Hz allow us to be relaxed and calm. Beta waves at 14-30 Hz allow our alert state. Theta waves at 4-8Hz allow us to enter into meditation, or deep relaxation and the beginnings of mental imagery. Finally, Delta waves at 1-3Hz is our deep, dreamless sleep state.

For purposes of this book, what you need to understand is that when there is an injury to brain tissue, even a minor one (from infection, head traumas), the area of trauma will naturally reduce its frequency generation. If this area is large enough, and the size can be very tiny to alter brain frequency generation, then another part of the brain will compensate and begin to generate those frequencies that are lacking as if the left arm tries to do more work while the right arm recovers.

The problem with this compensatory system is that brain tissue does not heal the way a fractured elbow would. The area of damage in the brain is akin to a rock hitting the windshield of your car window. Over time that minute fracture in your car window either starts to grow into a long crack affecting the entire functionality of the window or the crack stays contained but never disappears. The area of the brain that suffered the injury will do the same. The damaged area will either grow or it will go dormant. Other parts of the brain will take over in a compensatory function frequency wise. The problem with this over time is that each portion of the brain is designed to have a certain optimum frequency range. When the brain has to work overtime to compensate for another part of the brain that has "gone quiet" then this can fatigue the entire electrical system of the brain as if slowly draining a battery. This brain drain is another cause for keeping some unwary individuals stuck in their low energy trap!

Only by identifying the location of the frequency abnormalities in the brain and looking at these locations and ranges of frequencies generated in a brain from a compensatory (eyes open/standard EEG) as well as non-compensatory manner (eyes closed/qualitative EEG aka qEEG) can we assess whether the functionality of the brain in terms of its amplitude and volume of frequency generation is impacting the heart, thyroid and immune system leading to a chronic drain of energy in the patient.

The good news is that one need only have a qEEG done once a year. Neurofeedback helps to retrain the brain. Neurologists are not trained about qualitative EEGs sadly. It is a specialized form of training to take a qualitative EEG with eyes closed and eyes open. It has great advantages over an "eyes open" EEG done by allopathic doctors because only the qEEG shows what portions of the brain are trying to compensate for another region, which areas are not communicating well with each other and the depth of the problem.

Where can you get more information about qEEGs and neurofeedback? Go to ISNR, the International Society for Neurofeedback and Research (www.isnr.org). Bear in mind that most neurofeedback practitioners do not perform qEEGs before doing neurofeedback on a patient. I strongly believe this practice should change for the very reason that only the qEEG will show you with the utmost clarity the location of injury to the brain to avoid during neurofeedback.

In my own clinical practice with patients stuck in their low energy trap, if there has been any history of loss of consciousness from a fall, car accident, sports injury, and/or chronic ear infections as a child, or ear stents used, then I will strongly suggest to that patient that we have the qEEG and brain map done so that I can determine to what degree the "charge" in their brain has become so depleted that we are now looking at an electrical issue playing a significant role in keeping them in their low energy trap as opposed to or in conjunction with a hormonal and/or chemical or immune based issue.

The qEEG has explained why a patient of mine could not recover from low hormone function at the same rate as other patients. It showed her brain was fatiguing the entire body. In most cases, you can really boost immune system function and brain energy to support the whole body's recovery with neurofeedback once you know where to retrain the brain. At the same time, the brain map will also tell you the likely prognosis and stage of electrical fatigue of the brain. This explains why in some cases efforts to boost body function fall on deaf ears when it comes to springing someone out of their low energy trap. Their doctors focus on all the bodily functions but forget the significance of brain frequency function in keeping someone stuck in their low energy trap!

Here are some other examples of how the brain can impact the body and affect its outcome and prognosis. Some patients with "sensitive" digestive tracts suffer from food allergies and food sensitivities. Over time they find themselves becoming more and more reactive to more and more food. Many of these patients also experience neurological symptoms after eating certain food. They note brain fog, mental fatigue, increased agitation and irritability, racing or dark thoughts or have a short fuse after eating certain foods.

I have noticed that among those foods that create the most neurological symptoms for my patients are gluten and mold related foods such as peanut, corn (corn smut), oats (oat smut), raisins, cantaloupe, honeydew, grapes and strawberries. We refer to these foods in our clinics as "moldy" foods. Mold and mycotoxins seem to have more neurotoxic effects on susceptible brains, especially in those suffering from chronic inflammation, dysbiosis and food or other immune sensitivities.

This is an example of how a systemic condition, a food sensitivity to mold or mycotoxins can alter brain function. If this patient were to complain of fatigue and irritability to their allopathic doctor, most would suggest an anti-depressant or blame the thyroid! Most would not even think to look at that patient's diet as fuel for throwing off brain function!

I recently had a teenager complain of these exact symptoms and her general M.D. put her on an anti-depressant. When she returned to her doctor to say it wasn't working he changed her to another and another drug until she had tried four different anti-depressants before her mother brought her in to see us. That is when we discovered her extensive food triggers! She no longer needs any medications and her brain function and energy has returned.

Another patient helped her husband clean out their basement. After one day of that she was struck with brain fog and whole body fatigue to the point that she could barely take care of her two young children. Despite being in her 20's herself, her energy was completely drained. She advised me when she was in her home she now felt worse than when she left to do errands. A girlfriend visiting her suggested molds as a culprit because she said she now smelled something musty in the house while visiting. When we tested this young woman, sure enough, she had developed severe mold and mycotoxin sensitivities for which we treated and detoxified her. Her youthful vitality and mental sharpness returned despite having seen a dozen allopathic doctors all of whom suggest she take an anti-depressant as her only fix! This is an example of how a systemic (whole body) immune reaction can manifest with brain symptoms and fatigue which when undiagnosed, keeps you stuck in your low energy trap!

A third example was a woman in her sixties sent to me from her doctors to determine why she was not improving in her vitality despite her supplementation. We found food and environmental sensitivities. However, her fatigue and immune system function simply didn't rebound as it did with most patients receiving treatment. I suspected her brain had more to do with her whole body picture. This patient had normal EEGs yet her doctors scoffed at the idea of a qEEG. I ordered a qEEG. My qEEG technician ran the test and her brain map report showed deep and extensive alterations in her brain frequencies such that we could now see how her brain was impacting and limiting immune, thyroid and total vitality! Without extensive neurofeedback therapy, the degenerative processes in her brain, manifesting as reduced brain frequencies (like the draining of a battery) would result in her body not having the neurological support to assist in thyroid, heart and immune function. It now made sense why all the systemic support was not turning her condition around. Her brain was sinking her ship!

I have also seen cases where old brain traumas from childhood, sports head injuries and car accidents long forgotten after the body has healed, leave scars in the brain. Traumas to the brain that lead to the smallest scarring can also be a source for chronic headaches and migraine. They are the type that often do not respond to traditional prescription medications or de-sensitization to allergies and immune sensitivities. It's as if there is a hot spot in the brain that is susceptible to firing off. When it does, it triggers the headache/migraine attack, similar to how seizures occur. This is another example of how brain function triggers a whole body reaction.

Only recently with the emerging work of brave and brilliant research scientists and doctors is the momentum coming of age where the chemical and electrical workings of the brain are becoming available as part of one's evaluation in systemic (bodily) disorders. However, this is not the standard of care for allopathic medicine. In allopathic medicine many a seizure is never examined in the scope of a qEEG. Young or old, the patient is just put on seizure medications. The location in the brain where the seizure focus originated and its triggering causes is not examined or identified in the light of eliminating the source as a goal to eliminating the seizure. Instead the default mode is to keep the patient on seizure medications indefinitely!

With the advent of qEEGs and lab tests for brain chemistry, we can identify the location, severity of triggering focus and other parameters that speak to whether this patient can reverse their symptoms by addressing the triggering causes. A case in point was a young boy who suffered sudden onset seizure after a minor flu. Immediately his pediatrician recommended seizure medication. His parents were not happy with that suggestion and consulted our clinic. We found multiple triggers that would cause brain inflammation, including a weakened response to Epstein Barr, a virus that can enter the brain and cause inflammation. The child also tested low for the neurotransmitter GABA, which helps to calm the brain. When GABA is low or not absorbed well by neurons, seizures can become more frequent and severe.

Our treatment focus was to improve the child's GABA levels and eliminate sources of inflammation to both body and brain. The child could then undergo neurofeedback training, a system of brain bio-feedback to help heal and retrain the optimization of brain waves. In a year, the original seizure focus was eliminated. There was no evidence remaining in his brain to show a seizure focus! Of course his allopathic pediatrician was astonished because this type of fix does not happen with seizure medications! Had the child been put on seizure medication I guarantee you that his seizure focus would still be there, a dragon lying in dormancy but more than ready to spring forth with the next high fever or immune prompt. One has to wonder why this pediatrician did not call or meet with me about these results or refer me one of his challenging cases than to put his young patients on seizure meds for life!

With urine neurotransmitter testing, we can use the lab findings to track biochemical and metabolic progress in the brains of patients. We can compare a patient's symptomatic progress to what the patient is given to see if quantifiable changes in brain chemistry are working. An example is a patient suffering from anxiety and panic attacks. They frequently test low for GABA with urine neurotransmitter testing. Treatment to eliminate immune sensitivities to GABA, and boosting the patient's GABA levels will see the patient reporting feeling less anxious between panic attacks and the eventual reduction in frequency and severity of panic attacks. Working simultaneously on behavioral triggers will help to eliminate the brain entrainment that serves to trigger panic attacks. This is a far better solution that results in reduction and eventual elimination of a condition. The other option is allopathic medicine's masking the condition with ever increasing doses and types of prescription medication that lose their effect over time, permanently alter brain chemistry/receptor site information and cause the patient to be drug dependent indefinitely with no hope for cure.

The use of urine neurotransmitter testing will also stop the cycle of guesswork in prescribing drugs. Currently, if a prescription drug is reported by a patient to not work well, another is given in trial and error fashion without running any tests on brain chemistry. Why do we tolerate such haphazard treatment based upon guessing when clinically relevant tests for brain chemistry exist?

Worse yet, two or more prescription drugs are often combined. AARP conducted a study Published in 2005 entitled Prescription Drug Use Among Midlife and Older Americans to determine the number of prescription medications those 45 years and older were on. The number was four, taking four prescription drugs daily! (http://assets.aarp.org/rgcenter/health/rx_midlife_plus.pdf)

Did you know that no drug in America has ever been tested to be used together with another drug or over the counter medications as safe by the FDA? The drug is only tested by itself and not in combination with other medications. Who knows what the combined effects are.

Cutting edge medical practitioners now know that there is a direct correlation between urine excretion levels of neurotransmitters and clinical outcomes associated with symptoms. As a result, using an easy urine test can greatly assist in determining which neurotransmitter is relatively low or high and how effective one's course of treatment is in rebalancing one's brain chemistry, whether that treatment involves the use of a prescription drug or a natural compound or supplement.

Do you want to be treated by a doctor that says try this and see how you feel and if that doesn't work try that? We don't tolerate that with our car mechanic, electrician or plumber, so why do we tolerate that type of treatment with our bodies? Does a try this or that approach give you a sense of expertise in your doctor? Does that make you feel that he/she is working toward a solution to your problem or just placating symptoms and treating you like a lab rat?

Sadly the try this or that approach has become "mainstream" medicine as it is practiced today so long as the "do no harm" vow is not violated. It's high time the bar is raised for better medicine in conjunction with using state of the art lab testing. The block slowing the use of these labs has been resistance by insurance companies in covering only lab tests that focus mostly on disease diagnosis.

Cutting edge practitioners however know that NeuroScience Inc., a lab that runs urine neurotransmitter tests, is now approved with many significant insurance companies to measure your neurotransmitter excretions. They offer online teaching and certifications to health care practitioners about the efficacy and validity of urine neurotransmitter testing. Tell your doctor! The test is easy to do at home and once mailed, the results are emailed to your practitioner. Because NeuroScience Inc. is now covered by most insurance companies, they will process your lab through your insurance company first! Your doctor now has no excuse!

We at Immune Matrix have made urine neurotransmitter testing available to all our patients. The lab kit includes the cost of the medical consultation about your results. To order your neurotransmitter lab kit go to:

https://www.immunematrix.com/store

In summary, become aware of the factors affecting your brain that could be keeping you in your low energy trap, factors such as:

Low dopamine, GABA, and/or serotonin
Elevated glutamate
Elevated histamine
Elevated norepinephrine at the wrong time of day
Elevated dopamine at the wrong time of day
Brain inflammation (chronic hidden viral/bacterial infection, food sensitivities, toxic retention)
Old brain traumas having left a scar in your brain
Deficient brain nutrition, blood sugar metabolism
Lack of oxygenation, compromised brain circulation
Toxic retention in the brain
Immune sensitivities to mold/mycotoxins/environmental antigens

Then make sure you run a urine neurotransmitter test in the morning for general testing and before bed if you have sleep issues. Use this information to gauge your biochemistry and metabolism and work with a health care practitioner who regularly uses Neurosciences Inc. for best results.

PART 10 – WHAT ABOUT SLEEP

It goes without saying sleep plays a crucial role in one's ability to have energy during the day. Anything that interferes with the length of time and quality of your sleep will impact the quality of the energy you have during the day.

Solving the puzzle for what is keeping you from sleeping better and longer is as complicated as the puzzle for low energy itself. It has many contributing factors. I mention the subject of sleep because I want you to consider sleep as an issue and as a barometer of improvement as you overcome some of the issues mentioned in this book. The minimum goal should be to get at least six hours of good quality sleep and wake up feeling refreshed.

How do you know if you have sleep issues? You can break up the issue of sleep into those that can't fall asleep and those that can't stay asleep. Some individuals are plagued with both problems! A host of similar factors can affect one's ability to both fall asleep and stay asleep. For purposes of bringing to your attention possible culprits affecting your sleep I have listed certain key overlooked factors. This is by no means an in depth discussion on the subject. Consider any factors mentioned that could be affecting you as needing further investigation.

Pain:

Pain from structural issues such as a pinched nerve from disc compression to neuralgia's from Lyme disease or other neurological disorders can certainly affect one's ability to fall asleep and stay asleep.

Nutrient deficiencies caused by lifestyle, immune and digestive disorders and other chronic inflammatory conditions will also affect nerve function by altering biochemistry and thus sleep. When the body cannot repair the coating of nerves known as the myelin sheath, the nerve is more likely to fire off and therefore pain can be experienced more frequently and more severely when one's nutrient metabolism does not support the repair and regeneration of nerve tissue.

A little recognized source of pain is B vitamin deficiency. Certain B vitamin deficiencies are more common as we age as well as those suffering digestive and chronic inflammatory issues. Inflammation and digestive issues directly impact one's absorption of nutrients. For example, vitamin B1, B6 and B12, when deficient, can cause burning, stabbing pains and/or tingling in the feet and lower legs. The liver needs B vitamins to fuel its detoxification pathways. Therefore, it will compete for B vitamin stores to fuel its function. The liver is most active between the hours of midnight and 3 a.m. according to Chinese Medicine biorhythms. Thus one with B vitamin deficiencies could experience more restless sleep and neuralgias during this time, disturbing one's sleep. It could be mistaken for restless leg syndrome or symptoms from Lyme disease when in fact it is due to malabsorption and/or a deficiency in certain B vitamins.

It is interesting to note that one can show elevated blood levels of B vitamins and be functionally deficient in their absorption. This is a little known fact. What we have found in treating patients suffering from metabolic/immune issues is that if their immune system has become sensitized to a B vitamin and/or its metabolite, the body will be hindered in its absorption and usage of the B vitamin.

I originally found this occurring in autistic patients who also suffered genetic SNPs (defects) to their B vitamin and folate pathways. This slows their ability to process B vitamins and use folic acid. As a result, more metabolites build up in the blood and lymphatic tissue resulting in elevated B vitamin/folate lab results. Symptomatically the patient shows signs of B vitamin deficiency yet their lab results show elevated levels. When the patient is taken off their B vitamin/ folate supplementation, their ability to detoxify heavy metals and their neurological function suffers. The autistic child acts out with head banging, increased aggression and irritability.

When we desensitized the patient to the B vitamins and their metabolites, the patient's symptoms reversed. Their excretion levels of heavy metals resumed and their blood levels of B vitamin/folate returned to normal with no changes in supplementation. Therefore, elevated blood levels can either represent excessive intake or deficient utilization of the vitamin. Our computerized metabolic/immune pathway analysis helps us to determine which it is and treat accordingly.

A caveat to having one's immune system reactive to B vitamins/folate or their metabolites is that one can become reactive symptomatically to taking those supplements. When the immune system reacts to the B vitamin/folate or its metabolites you can experience symptoms ranging from racing heart, rashes, hyperactivity, irritability to blood sugar imbalances. B vitamin/folate absorption issues will directly impact one's brain chemistry because these vitamins are essential for the synthesis of many neurotransmitters for the brain. When certain neurotransmitters levels become low, the experience of pain can be heightened. Thus you have a mechanism for how increased severity of pain can then disturb one's sleep, all due to methylation/detoxification metabolic/immune triggers.

Another example of a nutrient deficiency increasing one's perception of nerve pain is Biotin. Biotin is a coenzyme in the vitamin B family. Its deficiency can cause the skin to become painful to touch along with tingling in the extremities. Nail ridges, thinning hair are also tip offs of biotin deficiency or malabsorption. Many individuals that are gluten free, individuals who cannot digest minerals from dark green leafy vegetables and have little tolerance for organ meats, eggs, and nuts become biotin deficient.

All these B vitamins by and large must come from our diet on a regular basis or we become deficient. Certain drugs can cause us to become deficient in B vitamins as can certain digestive disorders and chronic infections. Certain genetic variants inhibit one's ability to properly break down and/or manufacture B vitamins. Furthermore, having dysbiotic bacteria in one's colon further inhibits your ability to make B12 and other cofactors needed to repair nerve tissue. Therefore, it is best to work with a health care practitioner knowledgeable about the genetic SNPs of methylation and B vitamin synthesis and degradation to help determine what form of supplementation is best for your genes and metabolic/immune function to prevent adding to one's inflammation and to increase one's absorption of the vitamin.

Melatonin:

Melatonin is a hormone secreted by the pineal gland in our brain. As we age we seem to make less melatonin and sleep disturbances will result. Melatonin helps to stabilize our sleep cycles, protects our mitochondria and is a natural antioxidant. It is made from the amino acid tryptophan that many of us know is high in turkey. It is also made from the female hormone progesterone.

Deficiencies in the core nutrients needed to make melatonin can cause a deficiency in our melatonin synthesis. Women who stop ovulating due to peri-menopause or full menopause stop making progesterone. It is often at this time they begin to complain of difficulties falling asleep. Many health conditions that alter a woman's fertility cycle can also throw off her ovulation and thus interrupt her melatonin synthesis.

As of this writing, DiagnosTechs labs is currently working on adding salivary melatonin testing to their salivary cortisol panel to assess disturbances in the hypothalamus-pituitary-adrenal axis that can alter sleep patterns. Taking melatonin without determining if in fact your melatonin levels are low can cause morning fatigue from elevated melatonin levels and compound the problems with getting you out of your low energy trap.

With chronic infection in men or women, the body is more concerned with dealing with the infection than reproducing. Thus sex drive and fertility can become affected as can our sleep. We tend to assume that all our metabolic functions operate equally. However, infection and toxic retention exact a higher toll on the body consuming its nutrients resulting in reduced melatonin synthesis and thus reduced sleep.

Our pineal gland is often overlooked in the puzzle to improve one's sleep. It is a light sensitive organ even though it is located in the center of the brain, deep within the skull. Modern day lifestyle with electricity keeps us up well past sunset. This helps to throw off our melatonin biorhythm and synthesis. Therefore, sleeping with night lights or digital led lights in the bedroom will contribute to throwing off one's melatonin synthesis and biorhythm. Total darkness is advised to optimize one's melatonin synthesis in the bedroom.

I strongly suggest that before taking a melatonin supplement you run a salivary melatonin test to determine your melatonin biorhythm because excessive melatonin can contribute to fatigue. You can order melatonin test kits here: https://www.immunematrix.com/store

Liver Detoxification Issues:

Many patients we see struggle to digest their supplements, medications and food. The rate in which their liver breaks down and excretes toxins is limited by a combination of toxic retention overload and/or problems in the methylation pathway of the liver involved in how our body breaks down and excretes toxins. Many vitamins have to be converted in the liver to a bio-available form. When the liver is already stressed by genetic defects that slow the detoxification pathways of the liver, coupled by toxic retention pressing the body to step up its detoxification processes, the last thing to digest is often the very vitamin or medication we took. Like a conveyor belt backed up, multiple metabolic processes of the liver can suffer that fan out to affect brain, digestion, detoxification, hormone processing to name a few of the forty thousand metabolic processes the liver commands.

The subject of liver detoxification is a very complicated subject to simplify. It includes the subject of breaking down toxins, binding toxins for excretion, and using nutrients as biochemical building blocks and catalysts to fuel the entire process. Die-off poses a straw that breaks the camel's back for many a patient. If you are taking a product that is killing pathogens, then your liver has to process those pathogens for excretion. Sometimes the pathogens die off at a rate faster than your liver is capable of comfortably processing. If you experience sleep issues between the hours of midnight and 3:00 a.m., then you are most likely experiencing some type of stress to your liver which could either be overloaded with the process of detoxification or inefficient in some metabolic/immune manner.

Many a patient on an anti-fungal or Lyme disease program experiences problems with die-off, restless sleep and liver detoxification issues. All too many patients do not get sufficient detoxification support from their doctors while on their pathogen killing program. Thus the timing of your supplement program can help or hinder your liver detoxification and thus your sleep. If you are doing some type of cleansing program or detoxification and experience sleep disorders between midnight and 3:00 a.m., take it as a sign that you need additional detoxification support to assist your liver in processing toxins. Working with an experienced health care practitioner who knows the signs of die-off and can help your liver with the core nutrients it needs to process toxins especially at night can help you manage your pathogen killing program and spare your sleep.

Elevated Evening Brain Chemistry:

Some neurotransmitters help us to focus and be alert. These same neurotransmitters can hinder us from sleeping at night when their levels stay elevated. They keep our brains active when our bodies and brains need to enter into a relaxed state so that we can fall asleep and stay asleep. Norepinephrine and dopamine are two such neurotransmitters. We often see these neurotransmitters elevated in individuals having trouble falling asleep. Often the culprit is high glutamate levels caused by diet, or nutritional deficiencies preventing the proper breakdown and detoxification of these neurotransmitters. Other times another little known cause is due to having immune sensitivities to one's own neurotransmitters thus preventing the body from optimizing and balancing one's brain chemistry.

Doing a salivary neurotransmitter test before bed can be a helpful gauge to determine if your night time neurotransmitters are elevated and to what extent. You can order a test kit at:

https://www.immunematrix.com/store

PART 11 – BLOOD SUGAR

An inability to maintain even blood sugar levels throughout the night can make it difficult to fall asleep and stay asleep. Elevated blood sugar is over stimulating to the immune system and brain. It increases insulin and cortisol hormones that can increase inflammation in the body. Elevated blood sugar means more sugars in the blood available to feed pathogens in the body. This can cause a spike in symptoms stemming from dysbiosis in the gut, systemic yeast, candida and Lyme disease pathogens as well as chronic fatigue viral flares.

Low blood sugar while we sleep will hinder our body's ability to enter into sleep and to stay asleep. It hinders our body's ability to repair tissue. It throws off our brain chemistry. Our brain cells need glucose to function. Finally, low blood sugar can wake us up because our body signals that we are hungry.

There are many different reasons we experience problems with our blood sugar, both high and low. It often has a lot to do with what we've eaten throughout the day. How much protein we've eaten to help us maintain level blood sugar levels as well as the interplay of the hormones insulin and cortisol in affecting our night time blood sugar levels. Gut inflammation, dysbiosis, food allergies/sensitivities, insulin resistance, leptin resistance, immune sensitivities to cortisol, problems digesting protein, ghrelin imbalances, carbohydrates and/or fats and chronic inflammatory disorders are some common yet not commonly addressed causes for sleep disturbances.

Eating smaller portions every three hours along with protein and a digestive enzyme is an excellent lifestyle modification to promote even blood sugar throughout the day. It will ensure you enter your sleep stages with even blood sugar and hormone levels. Working with a knowledgeable health care provider that can look into the above mentioned imbalances can help you get to the bottom of why your sleep is keeping you stuck in your low energy trap.

PART 12 – ELEVATED EVENING CORTISOL

I've devoted the remainder of this book to discuss this most important hormone, cortisol. A red flag that elevated cortisol might be a culprit contributing to your inability to fall asleep and stay asleep would be that you are a night owl and find it easy to stay up late. You might feel tired but are too restless to sleep. You might even be more physically active at night when you should be ramping down. Elevated evening cortisol could be to blame. Read the chapter below on cortisol for more information.

Chapter 7

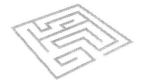

YOUR
INVISIBLE GLAND

The thyroid NEVER works independently of your adrenal glands. These glands are located above your kidneys. When the only focus is the thyroid as the culprit for fatigue, in that instance, your adrenal glands are "invisible" to your doctor. Rarely do allopathic doctors examine your adrenal gland function and its biorhythm. This is why I call your adrenal gland your "invisible" gland! Sadly, this oversight is routine!

This "invisible" glad (to your doctor) can mean a world of difference to you in regaining your energy and vitality. When sub-optimal adrenal function is addressed in conjunction with low thyroid or any other condition, you have the best chance of reversing not only the downward spiral to your energy, stamina and mental function but in reversing many degenerative, inflammatory, and metabolic related issues as well.

Why do I say this gland is largely invisible to allopathic physicians? With allopathic medicine's focus on disease diagnosis and treatment, its focus is narrow in view of the adrenal gland. Unless there is a disease classification that you now "qualify" for, just as in the case of diabetes, you will be told your adrenal glands are fine. Nothing could be more wrong! As with diabetes, you do not wake up one day suddenly with diabetes. Neither do you suddenly wake up one day with Cushing's, or Addison's disease from adrenal dysfunction. By that same token, you do not suddenly wake up with chronic suboptimal adrenal biorhythms!

YOUR ADRENAL BIORHYTHM

The adrenal glands are largely ignored by allopathic medicine unless a random blood test detects levels of cortisol (the hormone that the adrenal gland produces) that qualify the patient for a diagnosis of a disease such as Addison's disease (not enough cortisol) or Cushing's syndrome (too much cortisol production). If your random cortisol blood work is not elevated or low, you are told your adrenal glands are not diseased. Your allopathic doctor tells you your adrenals are fine. Nothing could be further from the truth.

The adrenal glands are small hormone-releasing organs located on top of each kidney. They have an outer portion called the cortex and an inner portion called the medulla, each with their own function. The cortex produces three types of hormones, two of which are key for your energy and stamina:

- a glucocorticoid hormone such as cortisol
- This hormone helps to regulate glucose, immune response, and helps the body respond to stress.
- a mineralocorticoid hormones such as aldosterone which regulates sodium and potassium balance, and the sex hormones, both male and female.

When the adrenal glands become "diseased", in the case of Addison's disease (also known as adrenocortical hypo-function, chronic adrenocortical insufficiency, or primary adrenal insufficiency) the adrenal glands do not produce enough cortisol. Addison's disease results from a dysfunction in the adrenal cortex. As a result, the cortex makes less of its hormone. (PubMed Health. A.D.A.M. Medical Encyclopedia. Atlanta (GA): A.D.A.M.; 2011)

Short of a disease of your adrenal glands, what can hamper adrenal gland function? Your adrenal glands will gradually produce less cortisol as a result of chronic stress, inflammation and infection. However, in the allopathic "disease" based view of health, nothing is done until your cortisol values "tank" below a certain agreed upon level to "qualify" you for the diagnosis of Addison's disease. This means that you can feel lousy, fatigued and even down right exhausted, have low immune function, suffer chronic infections, brain fatigue, hypoglycemia and hypo-secretion of other hormones, all because your adrenal glands are functioning sub-optimally, yet not "bad enough" to merit "allopathic medical attention" simply because they are not considered diseased!

Unless and until a patient reaches that dire stage of disease classification, nothing is said to the patient to even suggest that their adrenal gland function might be off. No one wakes up one day suddenly with diabetes or Addison's disease or Cushing's syndrome. The decline of adrenal function is a gradual process that our medical system is not taking heed to address unless that disease state is reached. It is a sad state of affairs to have to wait until one has developed a disease before taking action, especially when it's completely unnecessary!

Much can be done to reverse disease states and treat low energy in its early or even in its chronic stages when sub-optimal glandular function is caught and addressed. The key is to know your cortisol rhythm. It does not matter how long you have been suffering from fatigue. It also does not matter how long you have been on thyroid or other prescription medications. You cannot begin to improve your cortisol biorhythm until you know what it is.

What is a cortisol biorhythm? Your adrenal glands output cortisol (our stamina hormone) at different levels throughout the day in a pattern that is cyclical. This daily cortisol cycle is your biorhythm. Having a random blood test for cortisol completely misses the cortisol biorhythm because your blood is drawn only once and the time that it is drawn bears no correlation to your daily cortisol cycle.

Saliva testing is the only way to truly know your cortisol biorhythm.

Saliva testing for cortisol when done at specific times of the day will reflect your cortisol biorhythm. Why isn't saliva testing used in allopathic medicine? The simple answer is returning to the focus of allopathic medicine, that of detecting disease. If a one-time cortisol test happens to show high or low cortisol, then and only then is a disease suspected with respect to your adrenal glands. Allopathic medicine is not concerned about anything short of a diagnosis for Cushing's or Addison's when it comes to your adrenal glands by and large. That does not mean you are not fatigued. That does not mean you won't be heading toward the development of a disease. Why wait and suffer fatigue until you "qualify" for a disease diagnosis?

Saliva testing for hormones, and specifically for your cortisol biorhythm, is readily available. You spit into vials at specified times of the day and mail your results to the lab. With saliva testing readily available and affordably priced, why aren't allopathic doctors using this test regularly or at all? Besides the fact that allopathic medicine uses laboratory data for disease diagnosis, saliva testing had the historical criticism by doctors unaware of the advances in laboratory testing as to its significance and meaning as opposed to blood testing of cortisol.

In fact, salivary cortisol testing was officially recognized by The Endocrine Society (www.hormone.org) as a valid screening test for Cushing's Syndrome. Guidelines were published in the Journal of Clinical Endocrinology & Metabolism in 2008. (Patient Guide to the Diagnosis of Cushing's Syndrome, JCEM 2008 Vol 93) Nonetheless, too few insurance companies cover saliva cortisol testing. With that being said, there is little incentive for hospitals and private allopathic medical clinics to insist that these tests be used because the cost is out of pocket for the patient in many cases. However, the information is well worth the price. You will get answers you could not otherwise find with cortisol blood testing.

What distinguishes saliva testing from blood testing? Saliva testing's most significant advantage is that it reflects hormone levels that are present in tissue as opposed to the blood. How is that significant or important?

In the blood, proteins can bind the hormones and block the tissues from using them. Therefore, measuring hormones in the blood is deceptive because you don't see the percentage of hormones bound by proteins and therefore not available to be used by your tissues. This will therefore give a false sense of available hormones for the body to use because some or a significant percentage of your circulating hormones could in fact be bound to a protein (an antibody) that prevents the body from using it. Sadly, the saliva test is not main stream because the allopathic focus is to diagnose disease states.

Finding out the level of hormone that is available for your cells to use is critical. For cortisol, the best way to do that is with saliva testing. For thyroid, blood tests are available to quantify free circulating hormone levels as opposed to total hormone levels. Here's a classic example how low thyroid hormone diagnosis can be inaccurate because of lab testing.

When testing for thyroid hormone, your T3 (thyroid hormone) is tested on a standard blood panel. T3 is often referred to as Total T3. Blood levels of T3 reflect thyroid hormone bound as well as unbound to proteins (antibodies). Free T3 refers to the level of thyroid hormone not bound to protein/antibodies. The current standard of care for routine exams is to test by default only T3 aka Total T3.

If a patient's T3 (meaning total T3) is normal, the patient is told "your thyroid is fine", meaning your thyroid is making enough thyroid hormone. All the while, the patient is sitting there dog tired and may have all the classic signs of low thyroid function (cold extremities, thinning and loss of hair, loss of hair in the outer third of the eyebrows, slow digestion etc.) and wondering why. Had the doctor tested for "free T3, and looked for how much hormone was not bound to proteins and actually available for the tissues to use, they would likely have found low free T3 levels!

What is the sense of testing for T3 when one can test for **free** T3 (thyroid hormone that is free and not bound to a protein)? T3 testing is a test that should now be considered outdated as it gives the doctor and patient a false sense of security because higher levels of T3 are reported than are often actually available for your tissues to use. Testing for T3 misses the mark in finding cases of low free T3 and therefore misses the mark in finding out if you have insufficient thyroid hormone available for your tissues!

Many a patient is sent away told their thyroid hormone levels are fine based upon blood test results reflecting only "total T3" levels. The doctor never confirmed they had adequate levels of free T3. Many of these "normal" T3 patients have low free T3 and are not fine! I know, because I see this in our clinic all the time. This is a classic example of how a simple test that looks for your biorhythm or optimization of free hormone can be so helpful in confirming sub-optimal glandular/thyroid function.

A similar situation occurs in cortisol testing. Blood cortisol does not reflect the biorhythm of cortisol output during the day because it is taken only once in the day and randomly. Neither does blood testing of cortisol reflect the amount of cortisol available for the tissues to use, thus being "free" to be used by tissue. In addition, a person can have low cortisol production in the morning, normal cortisol levels at noon, and elevated cortisol in the afternoon and/or evening and/or at bedtime for example and be dog tired throughout the day, seek sweets for quick energy or that double-latte, gain belly fat and be wired and exhausted at bed time. Yet this person is told their cortisol is fine based upon a random timed blood cortisol test that happened to be taken when their blood cortisol level was normal and not high or low. The room for error is astronomical therefore in blood testing. Unless the blood is taken at the four critical times of the day to reflect one's cortisol biorhythm, it is useless in determining their cortisol output and biorhythm.

Few physicians have read the 2008 Endocrine Society's published guidelines recommending late night salivary cortisol testing for Cushing's syndrome. Despite this recommendation, no American hospital I know runs a saliva cortisol test yet alone a late night salivary cortisol test. Why not? If your doctor's head is in the sand and your insurance company cuts cost by denying you coverage for this exam, you need to wake up and get the test done yourself. It's a simple saliva test you can do in the privacy of your home. If you don't have access to the test from your health care practitioner, you can get one through Immune Matrix at https://www. immunematrix.com/store

There is a growing body of medicine called Functional Medicine, embraced by health care practitioners keenly interested in treating chronic illness as well as optimizing bodily functions prior to and in association with disease states. More and more allopathic doctors are embracing functional medicine in private practice where they have greater freedom to expand their tool box to include supplements and nutrients that optimize glandular function. One of the key tools in functional medicine is to quantify tissue levels of hormones and cortisol biorhythms. Saliva testing of cortisol is routinely performed by practitioners in the know in functional medicine.

HIGH OR LOW CORTISOL, DOES IT MATTER?

Once you run your saliva cortisol test how do you begin to understand the findings? Your biorhythm can be confusing to interpret because it can show high **or** low, high **and** low levels throughout the day. Both low and excessive cortisol secretion by your adrenal glands can cause you to feel low energy to various degrees. This is why you and your practitioner cannot determine what your cortisol values actually are based upon symptoms alone!

In addition, low thyroid function cannot generally be improved upon even with a prescription for exogenous thyroid (natural or synthetic) without also optimizing your adrenal function. The two glands are a part of a feedback loop where the glands communicate with each other and your brain! Therefore, if you do have issues with your thyroid gland then you absolutely must have a saliva cortisol test run.

Integrative and alternative medical practitioners have access to and many seek advanced training in the subtle nuances of optimizing cortisol biorhythms. They learn how to read salivary cortisol values, how to normalize them, and how to determine what is causing cortisol values to be out of range, either high or low.

Low energy can be due to high and/or low salivary cortisol values. You cannot tell whether you have high or low cortisol based simply upon how you feel. Take a look at the sample salivary cortisol report below.

Test	Description	Result		Ref Values	
TAP	Free Cortisol Rhythm				
TAP	Free Cortisol Rhythm				
	06:00 - 08:00 AM	17	Normal	13-24 nM	
	11:00 - 1:00 PM	32	Elevated	5-10 nM	
	04:00 - 05:00 PM	12	Elevated	3-8 nM	
	10:00 - Midnight	8	Elevated	1-4 nM	
	Cortisol Load:	69		23 - 42 nM	

The broad band that runs like a road through the graph reflects normal salivary cortisol ranges in a biorhythm that starts high in the morning and tapers down throughout the day. This person's salivary cortisol was dead center perfect in the morning, reflecting good strong adrenal function in the morning. Their cortisol however skyrocketed by noon because of the peak recorded at noon. The cortisol level began to taper down throughout the afternoon, but never came down to normal levels for the rest of the day or night because it was so elevated to begin with! This is how elevated cortisol can throw off your entire day!

This person could easily have a racing heart/thoughts, feel hungry all the time, even after eating a meal. They could feel wired and tired at night. They might crave sweets during the day and have intense evening/bedtime hunger followed by tossing and turning. This person's night time cortisol could prevent them from being able to relax sufficiently to get into deep sleep states. This person would gain weight easily because elevated cortisol elevates insulin. Their weight gain would tend to focus on the abdomen.

If this person had a blood test for cortisol during the day it would either be normal or elevated depending upon the time of day it was taken. The fluctuations and peaks for cortisol would be entirely missed. Had this individual's results shown low morning cortisol and elevated cortisol levels the rest of the day, a blood test for cortisol could have entirely different results and impressions depending upon the time of day the lab took the blood sample. In addition, as far as I am aware, most routine lab tests are done during 9 to 5 working hours and therefore one's bedtime cortisol would never be determined with a blood test. Can you now see how much information is missed entirely by a one-time random blood test that doesn't show you "available" and un-bound cortisol?!

HIGH CORTISOL

Let's go over some typical cortisol biorhythm examples.

One or More High Cortisol Values:

During those times when you have high cortisol, your insulin excretion can become excessive. This causes you to store fat immediately, even when you've eaten very little. Elevated cortisol causes you to become hungry, even shortly after eating. You seem to never feel satisfied. It becomes harder to maintain stable blood sugar levels with elevated cortisol and excessive insulin. Your blood sugar goes up, spiking after eating, along with your insulin. You store fat and then your blood sugar crashes and becomes low, causing hunger again. This cycle repeats daily like a roller coaster.

Elevated cortisol is also very damaging to the brain! Excessive cortisol lingers in the brain, killing brain cells, the ones located in the hippocampus. This leads to problems in thinking, focus, memory and logic. These damaging effects on the brain cause early onset pre-senile dementia which can begin to manifest in one's 50's. It is said that those that burn the candle at both ends, whose body is under a constant "stress response", for those who stay up late at night working on the computer, whose minds are overworked, overstimulated and under-rested, will have high cortisol values. These individuals will unknowingly be killing off their hippocampus cells until one day they reach a functional threshold of impairment and they begin to notice that their brain is not functioning as well. Once these specific brain cells die, their cumulative effect is to become easily distracted, challenged with short term memory and concentration issues.

Prolonged elevated cortisol is a huge risk factor leading to short term memory issues and early pre-senile dementia.

Many a busy executive in their 50's is already seeing the effects of having killed one too many brain cells due to a high stress lifestyle. Modern society applauds high achievers, the type 'A's, the selfless and the driven. However, the long term price these individuals pay is weight gain, fatigue, insomnia, blood sugar issues and early pre-senile dementia, to name a few. Is that the price you want to pay for material success?

Elevated cortisol also increases the body's overall level of inflammation because cortisol stimulates the immune system into action. It is like a bugle call that marshals the immune cells into action. The result is more inflammation derived from a heightened immune response. In the case of acute illness, a heightened immune response is a good thing because the cortisol activates your immune system to respond to a pathogenic threat of attack. In the case of chronic infection, the body cannot maintain elevated cortisol levels without consequences. Think about how difficult it would be for you to be blowing your bugle horn all day and all night! It would be exhausting. In time you could not keep up that pace. Your adrenal glands are no different. Over time they cannot respond to the constant stimulation that prompts them to make more cortisol.

Your adrenal glands will not only respond to your pushing yourself to burn the candle at both ends but to any perceived threat. For example, if you had to run from an attacker, your adrenal glands would immediately secrete a huge amount of cortisol in response to a perceived threat to allow you to access your sugar stores so that your muscles would have all the short term energy they needed to sprint from the threat. However, this sugar storage system in the body is quickly spent and you settle down into a lull or blood sugar crash after the event. At that time you need to nutritionally replenish your glucose storage as a result.

The same short term mobilization of your glucose stores happens when you have to push yourself physically to stay up late to finish a project or care for a sick child or do too many physical tasks during the span of your day (running yourself ragged). This response is also triggered when your body perceives it is under attack by infection, short or long term infection.

Depending upon how you react emotionally to your environment, your emotions also can prompt excessive cortisol output. For example, your boss, family members or spouse may be difficult to deal with. This creates frustration, anger, etc. which causes your body to react in a 'fight' mode where your body needs access to sugars so it can physically fight even though your brain has no intention of going fist to cuff. Nonetheless, your body has prepared you biologically for the perceived threat. Therefore, even though you bang your fist on the table and grit your teeth, your cortisol levels are shooting upward to prepare you for a fight.

Another example is perceived stress. Not everyone perceives a stressful situation in the same way. Some individuals hate last minute imposed projects and feel tremendous emotional anxiety, fear, etc. while another will thrive with the challenge. Other individuals will feel immediate anxiety at the thought of public speaking. How you react to people and interpret and react to your environment causes you to experience emotions (intentionally or unintentionally) which can cause your cortisol levels to become elevated. All these lifestyle factors must be considered if you expect to have any hope of living with balanced cortisol levels.

Sustained elevated cortisol depletes your immune system response much in the way that shouting "fire" repeatedly will elicit less and less of a reaction in people around you when the threat is not real. A depleted immune system will make you feel tired, keeping you in your low energy trap. As a result of repeated promptings of the adrenal glands to real or perceived infection, the immune response will also fatigue. Thus, elevated cortisol levels will fatigue your immune system and predispose you to more infections! Can you see the downward spiral making you feel more exhausted over time?

Elevated cortisol levels can also hinder thyroid function. Both the thyroid and adrenal glands communicate in what I call a relay system, a feedback loop that also includes your brain. Disconnect or damage this communication network system and you keep yourself locked in your low energy trap. Both the adrenal glands and the thyroid work to help you use your energy reserves. It makes sense if one gland is hyper-functioning, the other will ramp down its function to help maintain balance. Can you see how testing only for thyroid and not cortisol values leaves you in the dark on whether sub-optimal thyroid function is due to elevated cortisol levels? Can you also now understand that both the adrenal and thyroid glands have a direct impact on the energy we feel throughout our day?

You cannot determine by symptoms of fatigue alone who and what the culprit is or whether you have only one culprit. You can feel exhausted or wired and tired while your body is overstimulated just enough to keep you from getting restful sleep. These symptoms are often mistakenly attributed to low thyroid function alone when in fact they are more likely a combination of both and other factors mentioned in this book.

Since cortisol prompts your nervous system to respond in that fight or flight mode, the sympathetic nervous system in particular will go into fast action. Your heart rate will beat faster in the presence of more cortisol and your arteries will constrict in an effort to sustain blood flow to your heart so that you can "run" from this acute perceived threat. This is an inherent adaptive survival mode (running from the saber tooth tiger) that has helped man to survive for eons. The problem arises when sustained cortisol levels sustain arterial constriction, causing you to have a stress induced and now sustained elevation in blood pressure and heart rate. This is one simplistic mechanism how you develop hypertension from chronic stress.

Prolonged elevated cortisol contributes to the development of insulin resistance, Syndrome X.

Sustained elevated cortisol also increases your insulin output leading you to the development of insulin resistance aka Syndrome X. At least twenty five per cent of the American population suffers from Syndrome X reports the NIH. (Ford ES, Giles WH, Dietz WH (2002). "Prevalence of metabolic syndrome among US adults: findings from the third National Health and Nutrition Examination Survey". JAMA 287 (3): 356–359. doi:10.1001/jama.287.3.356. PMID 11790215) I suspect the percentage now is much higher gauging from the increase in obesity in the last eight years alone here in the United States.

How does insulin resistance/Syndrome X keep you in your low energy trap? Excessive insulin secretion causes the surface of your cells to ignore the prompting of insulin. Insulin is necessary to allow the transport of simple sugar molecules into the cell. When the signal of insulin is ramped up to the point that the cell membranes are constantly being bombarded by insulin, the cell membranes become overstimulated and shut down their sensitivity to the prompting of insulin. Imagine a family member running around you yelling fire, fire, when there is no fire. If you could not stop this person from shouting fire you tune them out. That is what your cells do when the volume and frequency of insulin's signal becomes excessive. It tunes it out. However, as a result, the cell becomes malnutritioned because unless it responds to the prompting of insulin and uses it to take in the simple sugar, it will be unable to have sufficient energy for cellular function. The consequence is the cell lacks energy and sends out signals to say it needs more glucose, making you hungry. You could even crave sugar!

This is how excessive output of insulin blocks your ability to use sugars. You will feel tired, exhausted and crave sugars for energy. A vicious cycle will start to form when you give into the carbohydrate cravings. More insulin is excreted than your cells can use and that continues to deaden and inhibit the ability of your cells to obtain the energy they are screaming out for as they continue to ignore the insulin signals they are being flooded with. Your cells will be unable to take in simple sugars to give them fuel. As a result, your circulating glucose levels rise. Instead of entering the cells the glucose stays in your bloodstream, elevating your blood sugar levels. Sustained elevated blood sugar further stimulates the body to excrete extra insulin to try to get your body to absorb this extra sugar. It also pushes you towards sustained insulin resistance, Syndrome X and the eventual development of diabetes.

The long term consequence of insulin resistance from elevated cortisol is that you have unabsorbed sugars circulating in your bloodstream. Unabsorbed sugars circulating in your blood can produce the following consequences, all of which are mechanisms that will keep you in your low energy trap:

1. The unabsorbed circulating sugars in your bloodstream make your body **acidic**. Acidic ph in your tissues impacts your energy in two ways. First, in order to use hormones and enzymes, they must be bathed in a specific ph range. When the range becomes more acidic, enzymes and hormones cannot function. Therefore, those metabolic processes that need enzymes to function (a majority

of bodily functions need enzymes) become less functional. Hormones become unavailable for use by tissues having become inactivated because of the lack of functional metabolic enzymes. The result is fatigue and slower metabolic processes.

2. The second major factor in having acidic terrain/tissues is that acidity is an open invitation for virus, bacteria, yeast, candida and other pathogens to come and live in your body. It invites infection and will weaken you and your immune system over time. The unabsorbed circulating sugars **feed pathogens** in your body making low grade and chronic viral/fungal/bacterial infections harder to eliminate. Many a doctor keeps a patient on antibiotics for months to years but never gets to the bottom of why their body "enables" them to exist. Acidity and excessive unabsorbed sugar in the bloodstream become an open door inviting chronic infection. Acidity needs to be eliminated to truly stop the infectious cycle which drains you and your immune system of vital energy, keeping you stuck in your low energy trap.

3. Unabsorbed circulating sugars form **AGE molecules** (advanced gylcation end products) in your tissues. These AGE molecules bind to your collagen, the substance in your tissue that allows you to have elastic and youthful skin. AGE molecules lead to connective tissue degradation and accelerated tissue aging, causing sagging, withered skin. Tissue degeneration inhibits proper nutrient absorption. Without proper nutrient absorption, synthesis of energy and cellular detoxification become hindered.

4. Unabsorbed sugars also circulate in the brain where they cause **brain inflammation**. These circulating sugars contribute to a form of insulin resistance in the brain that emerging science is calling "brain diabetes", the mal-absorption of glucose in brain cells. With any inflammation you will also see increases in cortisol which will kill brain cells in the hippocampus when sustained and elevated over time. Research is now looking at "brain diabetes" as a possible cause for Alzheimer's disease and dementia. If true,

the high stress executive has a double risk of brain damage from elevated cortisol and insulin resistance.

5. Insulin prompts the **storage of fat**. Elevated cortisol causes the development of more abdominal fat. This increases the output of the fat cell hormones because you now have more fat cells. In turn, these hormones cause further inflammation to your circulatory system. This leads to heart disease, stroke, arteriosclerosis, and elevated LDL cholesterol levels as well as more fat secreted hormones that prompt the body to store more fat! Fat is active metabolic tissue and yes it does secrete hormones that directly impact your energy, sugar metabolism, fat stores and inflammation. The more fat stores the more inflammation.

6. If the above were not bad enough, unabsorbed circulating sugars entrench your biochemistry into perpetuating the insulin resistance cycle prompting the constant secretion of insulin, fueling the cells to ignore its signal, preventing your use of simple sugars and keeping you mired in your low energy trap!

In summary, unabsorbed circulating sugars keep you locked in a cycle of perpetual elevated insulin resistance. Circulating sugars keep your tissues in an acidic state promoting infection and prolonging low grade infections that you become less efficient to eradicate. Elevation of fat and cortisol hormone levels cause you to store more fat. Acidic tissues also do not allow the proper use of enzymes and hormones and create molecules that degrade your tissues, increase free radical production damaging you cellular DNA, increase brain inflammation and cause a viscous cycle of creating more cortisol to fuel even more inflammation. All this puts your body on an endless round robin cycle of ever increasing fat accumulation, infection and hormonal imbalances. This is the metabolic web that locks you into your low energy trap.

The effects of elevated cortisol from increased insulin alone fans out to alter brain, liver, thyroid function, sugar metabolism, fat metabolism and storage, one's immune response, as well as skin and connective tissue regenerative abilities. Elevated cortisol can lead to increased skin sensitivity and purple colored stretch marks on the body as well as muscle weakness (often mistaken for signs of Lyme pathogens or their co-infectants).

Elevated cortisol, because of its inflammatory nature on the brain, will also heighten imbalances in brain chemistry. Elevated cortisol will make depression, anxiousness, and panic disorders worse. We have found this to be even more the case with Blood type A individuals, who already have very sensitive gut-brain connections.

Menstruating women can have their cycles thrown off by elevated cortisol to the extent that they no longer ovulate or menstruate regularly due to imbalances in the feedback loop between the adrenal glands, the ovaries and the pituitary gland in the brain. This is one mechanism of how stress induces infertility. The body is saying, when you have to run from the saber tooth tiger, who has time to get pregnant! It's Mother Nature's way of prioritizing biological function.

Excessive facial and body hair and decreased sex drive in men can occur when they have excessive cortisol. I like to remind my patients that when the body perceives stress, its concern is preservation, not sex! This is why libido can suffer with prolonged stress and/or maladaptation of the adrenal glands to chronic infection. Once the body returns to its state of balance, it's now safe to procreate and normal hormonal rhythms, desire and function return. Is elevated cortisol keeping you in your low energy trap, too tired to have interest in sex, too tired to put your all into your love life?

Does the Time of Day for Elevated Cortisol Matter?

How often and how much does cortisol need to be elevated to have a physiological impact on the body? Could elevated cortisol derail your energy, focus, biorhythms and metabolism? The answer is it does matter if your cortisol is elevated and it also matters how many times in the day your cortisol remains excessive. Elevated cortisol contributes to the maladaptive chemical stress response your body is producing that drives you to exhaustion and throws off other core metabolic functions. You have a cortisol biorhythm for a reason.

Looking at the cortisol biorhythm depicted in the above section entitled "High or Low Cortisol, Does It Matter?", your cortisol should be higher in the morning (within the wide band depicted) to get you going so you can do all the things the body needs to do in the morning.

As the day goes on, the body needs less and less stimulation so that we can begin to relax our cognitive, metabolic and digestive systems and enter into sleep, where healing and detoxification occur throughout the night. If we continue to output too much cortisol, it's like leaving the car parked in the garage but having a brick on the gas pedal while it's parked. It serves no purpose to reeve one's engine when you have nowhere to go.

If you start your day with elevated cortisol, it is as if your body is starting its day jumping out of bed and running to the train station. All internal systems are reeved. You can wake up hungry and tired because your blood sugar is low after fasting while sleeping. Yet elevated morning cortisol elevates insulin and reduces your ability to process carbohydrates. Fatigue and weight gain become your morning nemesis.

You can also experience a fast pulse and high blood pressure, anxiety, racing thoughts and even heart palpitations. The effect of reeving your body in the morning will inhibit digestion. When your body feels that it needs to run from a tiger, it doesn't want to digest food. It needs to fuel your muscles into action. The food you do eat in the morning when your cortisol is high will sit and ferment in your digestive system, causing acid reflux, bloating, nausea or a stagnant feeling. How many busy dashing executives complain of mid-morning indigestion? Elevated cortisol could be throwing off your digestion leading you to cellular malnutrition and insulin resistance. You end up feeling wired and tired in the morning.

With elevated morning cortisol you might feel as if you never got any rest at night. Actually, you didn't. With cortisol levels so high in your bloodstream, your body's ability to enter deep REM sleep is inhibited chemically. You'll feel a type of exhaustion that feels something like "if I could only get enough rest". This happens irrespective of how many hours you might sleep.

You also might also not want to eat breakfast with elevated morning cortisol. Having no appetite when your cortisol levels are high is your body's protective response. When your body perceives a threat, its response is "Who has time to eat?" Digestive juices shut down so your body can focus on escaping the perceived threat! Can you see how detrimental it is to start one's day running for a train?

If your salivary cortisol levels shoot through the roof at noon, your internal systems are running, running for that train again. Your heart beats faster than normal, blood pressure goes up and so does insulin. What you eat at lunch turns to fat easily and quickly because your body has pumped out extra insulin. In turn, you crave more carbohydrates to replenish your perceived dwindling glucose stores. Like most Americans, you then find yourself with a good appetite at lunch and eat too much in the way of carbohydrates for your metabolism and hormonal chemistry to metabolize and absorb. More insulin is secreted as a result of your carbohydrate laden lunch. Both your brain and your adrenal glands helped to elevate your insulin at lunch in a vain attempt to get your cells to start to absorb those sugars. Your brain cells are crying out for glucose for energy so you can focus and your body needs the fuel for sustained action, to escape that threat.

Despite your body's insulin signal, the cells resist using the insulin. They have over time tuned out listening to the prompts of insulin's signal. Your ability to absorb simple sugars to fuel your cells declines in direct proportion to your insulin resistance. You end up feeling tired, get brain fog and crave sugar!

Depending upon how long this cycle of elevated cortisol and elevated circulating insulin levels has been going on, your insulin resistance causes you to feel a crash in energy about an hour or two after lunch. The more carbohydrates you eat at lunch, the more you will feel fatigued after lunch. You respond by seeking a quick fix mid-afternoon. You eat more carbs, fruit, and/or caffeine. Some individuals might take stimulating supplements, B12, herbal adaptogens, even cortisol, thinking they are taking care of their adrenal glands. In fact, they had no idea they had elevated cortisol at this hour. For these individuals, they make their condition worse because these stimulants elevate their cortisol even higher!

In the late afternoon, before and around dinner, if your cortisol levels are high, you might actually feel highly productive and alert. You may get a lot done at this time of day, when cortisol levels are high, as opposed to when they are low or even normal because you will feel reeved. However, to maintain sustained elevated cortisol levels over time, your adrenal glands can become exhausted. It's like being on a treadmill at jogging speed all the time without rest, you and your adrenal gland will become fatigued and then exhausted.

Prolonged elevated cortisol will make you gain weight easily.

In addition, you will gain weight at those times of day when your cortisol is elevated because cortisol stimulates your body to make more insulin. If your cortisol is elevated around your dinner hour, and dinner is your biggest meal, then you will gain the most weight from this meal. You will also not feel as satisfied from dinner because the extra insulin will make you feel hungry, even after a big meal. How much carbohydrate you eat coupled with the time of day your cortisol is elevated will fuel insulin resistance and keep you in your low energy trap! This is why you absolutely need to know your cortisol rhythm!

If your cortisol levels climb in the evening and remain elevated into the night, you can feel wired yet tired. You find it hard to relax at night. Your higher energy level at night will make it difficult for you to fall asleep. You might stay active and do too much too late into the evening to prevent you from ramping your energy down to get into that restful sleep inducing state.

You can also find yourself getting hungry after dinner with elevated cortisol levels. You may even feel hungry late night, before bed despite having had a good dinner. You might crave carbohydrates, like cereal or other refined carbohydrates as a snack for quick energy before bed. If you indulge, you will surely gain weight at this hour of eating.

With elevated evening cortisol levels, you might feel very alert and decide to use this energy to continue to do things like watch TV, play videogames, and "do" too much when you should be ramping down to rest. The result is, you stay up later, have a harder time falling asleep, experience a less restful sleep as well as fewer hours of sleep. The end result, less rest and rejuvenation and less time your body has to detoxify and regenerate. All the while, all the factors that occur with elevated cortisol continue to wreak havoc on your brain, your energy, your hormone production, immune system function, tissues repair and regeneration, as well as digestive function and detoxification.

Can you now comprehend when your doctor fails to order a saliva cortisol test, it's as if your adrenal glands were "invisible"? Can you now understand cortisol's significant effect upon the body and its proper biorhythm throughout the day as significant and integral to proper health? When your adrenal glands are "invisible" and you and your health care practitioner has no idea what your cortisol biorhythm is, you and your health care practitioner have no idea how your adrenal glands are impacting your body to hinder or inhibit your energy production and usage as well as so many other essential metabolic processes.

In summary, here are a few additional examples of the effects cortisol has on the body:

1. Elevated cortisol stimulates excessive insulin secretion. Elevated insulin levels lead to and cause the development of insulin resistance/syndrome X, and inhibit proper carbohydrate metabolism, resulting in the telltale signs of fatigue after meals containing carbohydrates in direct proportion to your level of insulin resistance and the amount of carbohydrates eaten.

2. Elevated cortisol causes you to gain fat mass despite cutting down on what you eat (especially weight along the waistline).

3. Elevated cortisol will throw off your sleep cycle and diminish the quality of your rest. Less sleep means you can begin to develop leptin resistance, a hormone that controls appetite and fat storage. You will want to eat more and reap less energy from the food you eat when you are leptin resistant! This is how one hormone imbalance impacts and causes other hormone imbalances.

4. Elevated cortisol will cause you to feel hungry all the time, even after you've eaten a full meal. You will never feel satisfied. Again, leptin resistance may be a significant contributing factor to your constant state of hunger as with insulin resistance.

5. Elevated cortisol fuels inflammation in the body. This causes brain inflammation and brain cell death (hippocampus brain cells) accelerating brain aging and cognitive disorders. Inflammation also degrades cell wall membranes, preventing tissue healing and nutrient absorption. Your cells starve for energy while the nutrients circulate in your blood stream and feed pathogens.

6. Elevated cortisol tells your body to be on high alert, that you need to run to escape the perceived threat, and thus elevates blood pressure.

7. Elevated cortisol predisposes you to chronic pathogenic infections requiring constant medications to control, draining your body of its immune and energy reserves.

8. Elevated cortisol causes your energy to lag, to feel exhausted with low stamina and have slow or little recovery after physical exertion, activity or stress.

9. Elevated cortisol causes accelerated degeneration of connective tissue and collagen.

10. Elevated cortisol exhausts your immune response and therefore you!

11. Elevated cortisol exhausts your adrenal glands. They cannot keep up with the constant treadmill of stress your body's chemical signals send them.

Another Cause:

Sometimes the cause for sustained elevated cortisol is not the result of maladaptation of the adrenal glands but *depletion of choline reserves* in the body. Choline is needed by the body as a precursor to make brain hormones aka neurotransmitters essential for brain function. It is also an essential nutrient for muscle control as well as for the repair of the outer covering of nerves (the myelin sheath). Choline is essential for cell membrane repair, forming an integral component of the phospholipid membranes in our tissues. When we cannot replenish our tissue choline our tissues will become lax and aged.

We must get our choline stores from the food we eat. Choline comes from fatty meats and eggs. Most of us are deficient in choline due to our efforts to manage our cholesterol by reducing our consumption of meat and eggs. The Dietary Reference Intake (DRI) is a system of nutritional recommendations from the Institute of Medicine (IOM) of the U.S. National Academy of Sciences. The DRI recommends that an adequate intake (AI) of choline is 425 milligrams per day for adult women, and higher for pregnant and breastfeeding women. The AI for adult men is recommended at 550 mg/day. There are also AIs for children and teens.

Below is a list of animal and food sources for Choline (mg): (http://en.wikipedia.org/wiki/Choline)

- 5 ounces (142 g) raw beef liver 473mg
- Large hardboiled egg 113mg
- Half a pound (227 g) cod fish 190mg
- Half a pound of chicken 150mg
- Quart of milk, 1% fat 173mg
- A gram soy lecithin 30mg
- 100 grams of Soybeans dry 116mg
- A pound (454 grams) of cauliflower 177mg
- A pound of spinach 113mg
- A cup of wheat germ 202mg
- Two cups (0.47 liters) firm tofu 142mg
- Two cups of cooked kidney beans 108mg
- A cup of uncooked quinoa 119mg
- A cup of uncooked amaranth 135mg
- A grapefruit 19mg
- Three cups (710 cc) cooked brown rice 54mg
- A cup (143 g) of almonds 74mg

Examining the food sources for choline, you have to eat quite a bit of certain foods to get adequate amounts of choline. Looking at the food list above that simply is not practical. You need to eat more of these foods when one's cortisol values are up and your need for choline is enhanced. It's no wonder that we are often deficient in our choline intake.

Besides a low dietary intake of high choline foods, how else can we become choline deficient? With acute and chronic stress your need for choline will increase for the very reason that choline is an essential precursor molecule for the synthesis of phosphotidylserine. Phosphotidylserine is a molecule that helps to break down cortisol so that it can be excreted by the body. All hormones are made and then degraded and detoxified by the body. When your body cannot make enough of this molecule, your ability to reduce excessive cortisol by detoxifying it is limited and therefore another mechanism for elevated cortisol is a diet deficient in choline.

This is why when elevated levels of cortisol are seen, the supplement phosphotidylserine is often given to be taken at the time of day when your salivary cortisol level is high. The elevated cortisol can quickly exhaust your choline reserves causing your cortisol levels to remain elevated long after the perceived threat that prompted the initial elevation in cortisol is gone. This is a prime example of how diet and lifestyle interact to keep you in your low energy trap!

A cheaper and just as effective source of phosphotidylserine would be to take lecithin in liquid or granule form daily. I sprinkle a heaping tablespoon of the granules over my salad, cottage cheese, hide it in my warm soups, and add it to smoothies. Since it is a fat, it will go rancid; therefore, store it refrigerated. Since it is a fat, it mixes better with oil based foods, warm foods, and things you can blend like a smoothie as opposed to putting it in your water (not advised) where it will not blend or dissolve.

In summary and as a last caveat to the issue of elevated cortisol, be sure to interpret your result in light of your recent (last 3 month) lifestyle experiences for the possible cause as to why your cortisol values were high at that time of day. There is always an exogenous (outside) trigger such as infection, emotional stressor, or lifestyle habit stressing the body and prompting the elevation of cortisol. The more serious and prolonged the stressor, the more likely cortisol values will stay elevated long after the trigger is gone.

LOW CORTISOL LEVELS

How Does One Develop Low Cortisol Levels?

Your adrenal glands respond to stress initially by making more cortisol. This helps your body mobilize and use sugars for quick response (to run from that saber tooth tiger) and to marshal your immune cells for the perceived pathogenic attack your body is under.

The problem arises when the "stressor" becomes chronic. What are chronic stressors? Chronic low grade infections can weaken the adrenal glands. These infections can originate from the gums and digestive tract, dysbiotic bacteria/fungus/yeast/candida. Infections both acute and chronic, from virus or other stealthy bacteria, spirochetes, yeast and/or candida all take their toll in over stimulating the adrenal glands. Emotional stressors such as work stress or family and relational stress can tax your adrenal stamina. Daily lifestyle habits that prevent your body from experiencing sufficient down time, rest, relaxation, detoxification and quality sleep will wear you and your adrenal glands down. Finally, nutritional deficiencies or excesses can hinder proper adrenal function, contributing to low cortisol output.

When the stressor is prolonged, your adrenal glands form a hormonal habitual response to the stressor just as you form a reactive habitual response to what you do when you perceive stress. Your hormonal habitual stress response becomes a part of your cortisol biorhythm long after the need for the extra cortisol is gone. Your hormonal habitual stressor response causes your adrenal glands to continue to secrete cortisol at a higher level as a result of prolonged stress, long after that event is over. The result is the eventual fatigue of your adrenal glands.

When the "stressor" is gone (sick child better, work deadline done, acute stage of infection now in recovery) your adrenal glands are less likely to revert to normal levels of cortisol output the longer they were "pressed by stress". This is because in part, your adrenal glands habituated to the stressor and have now altered their biorhythm to secrete excessive amounts of cortisol to help your body deal with the stressor. Unfortunately, the continued excessive production of cortisol becomes your habituated response to any stressor now, even minor stress. In addition, it takes the adrenal glands longer to "down-regulate" after prolonged stress because of this "habituation".

As your body wears down from the constant presence of taxing stressors, other hormonal systems also become less functional. Lower production and secretion of other hormones can result as well. Another byproduct of exposure to a prolonged stressor will result in less production of a hormone precursor that your adrenal glands need in order to make cortisol called DHEA (Dehydroepiandrosterone). A deficiency of this hormone prevents your body from optimizing hormone synthesis, especially cortisol. This precursor hormone is so important that it is included in the salivary cortisol hormone panel by Diagnos-Techs™. To expect to be able to increase your cortisol output when you have low DHEA is to expect to increase one's savings account but never deposit money into the bank! It just won't happen.

Another byproduct of stress is it makes you acidic! Stress increases your need for alkaline minerals to help neutralize the acid your body creates from the stressor. In addition, the more acidic you become, the less you are able to use your hormones, including cortisol because hormones have to operate within a certain ph range. Becoming acidic causes you to be unable to use what little hormone your exhausted adrenal glands do make! That goes for every hormone in your body! Stress therefore creates a vicious cycle of depleted hormone synthesis and usage.

Chronic stress can lower cortisol levels
at any or all times of the day.

When can we experience low cortisol levels? Low cortisol values can occur at any time of day. They can occur just in the morning, or at noon, before dinner or at bedtime or all of the above! Over time, the entire cortisol rhythm will become low as adrenal gland function declines from the stressors, leaving you with low cortisol throughout the entire day.

What are the consequences of low cortisol values? Initially what commonly occurs is that the morning cortisol level will be low. Often this occurs as a result of elevated night cortisol and/or low DHEA values. You wake up feeling unrested and tired. Sleeping in will not solve the problem. In fact, even when you sleep in you do not wake up any more refreshed or energized!

In addition, depending upon how low your morning cortisol level actually is, in addition to feeling tired and/or exhausted, your body will not use carbohydrates well. The reason for this is that you need sufficient amounts of cortisol to prompt the output of insulin. As a result, you may have no appetite for breakfast when your morning cortisol is low and what food you do eat feels as if it sits in your digestive tract. Your brain could feel groggy or slow and not alert in the morning. Muscle movement and strength will be low because your muscle cells need energy from glucose. With low cortisol you have low immune function and slower communication with systems affecting your metabolism. Therefore, thyroid function can and will also suffer. Can you see the downward spiral that just low morning cortisol causes to keep you in your low energy trap?

When your morning cortisol is low you might crave a stimulant such as caffeine to boost your adrenal glands into making more cortisol! However, as the adrenal glands go from a state of fatigue to chronic fatigue to exhaustion, the adrenal glands will be less responsive to stimulants, nutritionally or nutraceutically! When you do drink your coffee, you will notice that it's less effective in boosting your energy and you will be tempted to drink more than one cup. Soon you will have to down a pot of coffee to get going. When that fails to work, many resort to expreso drinks.

When your cortisol is low at the lunch or dinner hour, you will feel like this is your low energy time of day. You are more awake now than when you woke up but your energy is lagging. Motivation is often low. You need to push yourself to get things done because your energy just isn't there. With lunch and dinner, you tend to crave carbohydrates in an effort to get a quick pick me up. You might even crave sweets after your meal. Your food doesn't seem to give you the energy you need.

If you've had a low level of cortisol for a while at the lunch or dinner hour, you may notice that when you do eat carbohydrates at lunch or dinner in the form of sandwiches, pasta or rice dishes, you feel tired after your meal and crave a nap. You might have already started to reduce the volume of carbohydrates you eat at lunch or dinner but you notice you still feel that lull in your energy, just not as badly. You compensate by taking in caffeine, high glycemic fruits (banana) or sugary snacks (cookies, pastries) to boost your energy which never quite comes up to your expectations. You may notice you are gaining weight easier too!

If your low cortisol rhythm occurs at dinner (and sometimes for those with low cortisol at noon), you will often feel a mid-afternoon slump in energy. This can occur anywhere from 2:00 p.m. to 4:00 p.m. Mid-afternoon becomes your least productive time of day and the most likely time for you to crave that carbohydrate snack or caffeine boost!

With low cortisol, your entire metabolism slows down. Brain focus and speed can suffer as can drive and stamina to accomplish tasks. You are the most sensitive to developing insulin resistance when your cortisol level is low. In addition, eating carbohydrates at the time of day when your cortisol levels are low can make your adrenal glands weaker yet. You will crave carbohydrates as energy but if you indulge in more carbohydrates when your cortisol is low you foster insulin resistance and weaken your adrenal glands even more!

Low cortisol output also slows your digestion. Food might feel like it's not moving through your digestive system and you may have little appetite as a result. You might not feel hunger when you need to. Instead you will more likely feel fatigued. When you do eat, the fatigue will be alleviated to an extent with a small snack to pump up your blood sugar. Eating more tires you, yet a small amount will pick your energy up.

Accordingly, low cortisol can cause you to go into a reactive hypoglycemic state where your blood sugar drops along with your energy until you eat something. You often fail to feel a normal hunger response. It's easy to attribute the fatigue brought on by low blood sugar stemming from low cortisol, to something else (low thyroid, chronic fatigue virus, Lyme disease etc.) when in fact it has been brought on by low cortisol. This can be entirely missed by your health care practitioner if a saliva cortisol test is not run.

With constant low energy, you find it increasingly more difficult to care for yourself. Cooking good healthy food becomes harder and harder as you have to muster the energy to shop as well as prepare the food and clean up. You may opt instead for quick fixes, microwaved meals and carbohydrate dominant foods. These foods are low in nutrition and increase your insulin resistance. They are higher in carbohydrates and will weaken your adrenal glands further.

You know you also need to move your body and get some exercise but you can't seem to muster the energy to do it. If you do, you find the next day you are even more tired! Some of you with very low cortisol output will be exhausted simply from the effort it takes to shop for your groceries! You can't seem to recover from the exertion, any exertion.

You may also find that you have chronic lingering infections. Infections such as candidiasis, gum irritations, chronic or recurrent sinus infections, more frequent colds, all common with low cortisol. You may also suffer from more aches and pains, muscle aches and joint pains or nagging swollen lymph nodes.

In the later stages of adrenal exhaustion, your cortisol values will remain low well into the night. This makes you feel drained throughout the evening. You have a difficult time doing essential lifestyle tasks. You might find you have to let tasks slip now to cope and get through your evening. You go to bed feeling drained and exhausted but can't seem to get into a deep sleep. Sleep may be light and restless and definitely not rejuvenating.

At this stage many people decide to go see their doctor. A blood test is run only for thyroid. Sometimes "a" serum cortisol value is also run. In most cases, the person is told it's their thyroid. Your thyroid may be contributing to the problem but by now you can see that the entire biorhythm of your adrenal gland is being ignored. Thus your "invisible gland" receives no attention or care and therefore no hope for rejuvenation.

Whether you have high cortisol or low cortisol or both, it matters considerably to your stamina, hunger levels, feelings of stress, restlessness, ability to maintain proper blood sugar levels and ability to have restful sleep. As you can now begin to understand, you cannot determine what and where your cortisol values are during the day by symptoms alone.

The adrenal glands do not function independently from the thyroid gland, your sugar metabolism or immune function. It's a delicate balance with one system affecting another. To treat thyroid alone is like fixing the screen on one window pane of a house to stop the flies from coming in and ignoring other broken window panes! You will get some relief but it doesn't fix the problem.

You can also begin to see why measuring your cortisol via blood misses the mark in letting you know what your cortisol rhythm is throughout the day. Your cortisol output affects your entire metabolism as the day progresses and has significant impact during key points of the day on many biological functions. Knowing when your cortisol is low or high is essential for knowing how and *when* to treat it. Symptoms alone won't tell you what your cortisol values are because one can feel tired and have elevated cortisol levels just as easily as low cortisol values!

Treatment For Low Cortisol

The treatment for low cortisol output versus excessive cortisol output is entirely different from each other. The confusing aspect is symptoms of fatigue and exhaustion can be the same. As we described above, the causes for low cortisol versus excessive cortisol output are different. Understanding how you develop low or high cortisol is essential for successful treatment.

Sadly, many health care practitioners not only ignore this gland, but treat adrenal "issues" based upon "obvious" clinical symptoms of exhaustion without ever ordering a salivary cortisol test. Do not let your health care provider give you cortisol boosting supplements without running a salivary cortisol test. If you do, you run the risk in a short period of time of developing elevated cortisol and you won't feel it or realize it initially. In addition, those practitioners who do not use the salivary cortisol test often have you taking your cortisol boosting supplement at the wrong time of day. This risks throwing off your entire cortisol rhythm or elevating otherwise normal cortisol. It's sloppy medicine, so don't allow it. You need to know what not to do in case your health care provider is making this mistake with you! You have only the risk of never optimizing your cortisol rhythm or making it worse!

What Not To Do:

The medical knee jerk reaction upon discovering a low "serum" (blood test) for cortisol is to put you on cortisol to raise your level of cortisol. Why is that a bad thing sometimes? It's a bad thing for two reasons. First of all, giving your body cortisol tells your adrenal glands they don't have to make cortisol because there is an exogenous (outside) source for it. It's called a "negative feedback loop". Exogenous cortisol signals the adrenal glands to stop making more. The longer you take cortisol the lazier your adrenal glands will become as they perceive the presence of cortisol so they do not need to make anymore.

> *Exogenous cortisol is a temporary crutch that with long term use will weaken your adrenal glands.*

Exogenous cortisol makes you dependent upon outside sources of cortisol to continue to thrive. Your adrenal glands will atrophy. Getting them to make optimal levels once you stop taking the exogenous cortisol will take longer. Big Pharma and allopathic medicine loves the fact you are now on something that reaps profits for them long term. Besides, their attitude is it doesn't harm you so what is the harm in becoming dependent on it when you 'apparently' need it. It's a prescription for life! The problem is they know better. Yes it takes more effort to rebuild your adrenal gland function but it's so much faster, easier and profitable to just give you a prescription for cortisol and keep you dependent indefinitely. That attitude isn't helping you solve your problem. It only keeps you stuck in your low energy trap. Your adrenal glands atrophy and more often than not your body becomes resistant to this exogenous cortisol!

Is there ever a time when exogenous cortisol is justified? In some cases, when the patient is so exhausted by active chronic infection (Lyme disease for example) or chronic viral infections affecting the thyroid (Epstein Barr for example), and salivary cortisol levels are so low, coupled with symptoms of exhaustion, short term exogenous cortisol will help. It will give the patient that "crutch" to boost immune function, improve sugar metabolism, blood sugar and brain function to carry them through their other treatment therapies.

The problem arises when a majority of these doctors neglect to have a protocol to "wean" the patient off of exogenous cortisol and begin to help the adrenals function on their own. I rarely see this done by allopathic doctors. I see so much medical complacency and contentment in relying upon insurance covered prescriptions. This creates a dependency and weakens your adrenal glands. Rather than work with the patient, monitor their cortisol output and seek to strengthen the adrenal glands by proper supplementation, the patient is simply given cortisol. This is not in your highest and best interest in the long run.

The second reason exogenous cortisol can be problematic is that it is generally prescribed without any reference to time of day for taking it. If your salivary cortisol values are high in the morning, and you are told or just happen to take your cortisol or cortisol promoting supplement in the morning, along with your other supplements, your cortisol level will increase even more! You 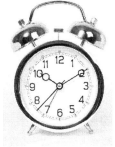 would have entirely missed the mark on boosting low cortisol at another time of day. Furthermore, you could easily elevate a normal cortisol value by taking your prescription/cortisol supplement when your cortisol was normal or worse, already elevated!

For example, if salivary cortisol is low at 4p.m., and normal the rest of the day, taking cortisol in the morning can cause an elevation of morning cortisol. Furthermore, the cortisol level will not generally increase six hours after taking a supplement when you need to boost cortisol output at 4 p.m. The time of day you take your cortisol boosting supplement is crucial.

If your health care provider has made no provision to correlate the time of day you take your cortisol to when your cortisol values actually are low, then not only are you not using this exogenous cortisol effectively, your health care provider could be causing you harm by allowing you to derail your cortisol biorhythm. Elevation of otherwise normal values is the risk while simultaneously not improving low values.

Are you any safer taking supplements advertised for adrenal function? No matter what you take to increase cortisol output and to improve adrenal gland strength, the best supplement can still backfire if taken at the wrong time of day. Taking ginseng, a Chinese herbal formula, a homeopathic, herbal and/or neutraceutical adaptogens at the wrong time of day can overstimulate the adrenal glands when cortisol output is normal or already elevated!

The same rule of thumb applies whenever you attempt to increase otherwise low cortisol numbers. Take your adrenal supplements at the time of day when your cortisol level is low in order to best increase adrenal function.

If you have low cortisol levels, you really should work with an experienced health care practitioner to ensure that your adrenal glands actually become stronger if you want to have any hope of walking out of this valley of fatigue. Too many patients suffer for years not realizing that they could improve their cortisol values or think their health care practitioner has done all that can be done! If you do not also address the causes for low cortisol, you and your health care practitioner will not be effective in reversing chronic low adrenal function. Your endless cycle of fatigue will keep you in your low energy trap.

Not everyone is created equal in their ability to tolerate herbs, supplements and tinctures. An experienced health care practitioner knows which supplements, herbs, and tinctures will improve cortisol values and how long that usually will take. They will also use the salivary cortisol test as your initial and follow up assessment. Furthermore, certain blood types have a more difficult time with certain types of remedies. Therefore, working with an experienced practitioner, one who knows how to get results with different metabolisms, blood types, liver detoxification pathway limitations and supplement intolerances will optimize and shorten your recovery time.

At Immune Matrix clinics, we distinguish each patient's ability to detoxify and metabolize specific nutrients. This helps us to determine their metabolic/immune intolerances as well as their ability to respond to prescribed supplements. We also look at food sensitivities that impact one's ability to digest supplements and process carbohydrates, as this will affect adrenal function. Furthermore, we use the latest research to tailor your specific blood chemistry, immune sensitivities, detoxification pathways and digestive limitations to determine the adrenal formula that best suits your specific adrenal biorhythm. For example, the blood type A is the least able to digest and metabolize certain supplements. Few practitioners appreciate this significant find or know how to help a chronically ill blood type A patient handle supplements, especially if their livers have challenges with methylation.

What Can YOU Do to Improve Low Adrenal Function?

There is much you can do by way of lifestyle habits that can either help or hinder your cortisol rhythm. When your cortisol levels are low, your carbohydrate metabolism and your ability to use simple sugars is easily hindered. You are at greater risk of developing insulin resistance/Syndrome X. What you must do is restrict the amount of carbohydrates you eat at the meal when your cortisol is low. The more carbohydrates you eat, the more you stress your adrenal glands. Therefore, you must parcel out the amount of carbohydrates you eat when your cortisol is low to avoid aggravating sugar metabolism issues and the possible creation and/or aggravation of insulin resistance.

A rule of thumb is to observe how tired you are after a meal containing any carbohydrate, complex or simple/refined, such as potato/rice/bread/legumes or root vegetables. Keep reducing the amount of carbohydrate you eat at that meal until you no long feel fatigued within an hour or two after your meal. Try to routinely rate your fatigue on a scale of 1-10 with

10 being exhausted and having to nap to a 1, meaning negligible fatigue. In many cases with low cortisol, one has to omit carbohydrates at that meal to prevent post meal fatigue. As your adrenal glands strengthen, your carbohydrate metabolism should improve as will your insulin resistance and post meal fatigue.

Improving the breakdown of your food will help to ensure more nutrients are available for absorption by your cells. The best way to do this, and the safest way is to take a digestive enzyme as soon as you start to eat. Immune Matrix patients are given their proprietary digestive enzyme called "Ultimate Digestion" available online at www.immunematrix. com. It assists in breaking down fiber, carbohydrates, protein, fats, food additives and gluten byproducts. The last two functions are lacking in most enzyme blends. I do not recommend eating gluten but it was added to the enzyme blend because it sneaks into many products unknown to the public. It helps in the breakdown of the gluten proteins but will not prevent the inflammatory effects and gene activation from gluten, gliadin and glutenin.

Taking a digestive enzyme will not inhibit the production of your own digestive enzymes. For those suffering with energy depletion, taking a digestive enzyme can be one of the best energy saving things you can do for your body. The reason digestive enzymes help save energy is that the synthesis of enzymes is "the" most taxing metabolic function the body does. All metabolic processes of the body are run via enzymes. Therefore, the body is constantly under pressure to keep up with enzyme production. Supplying the body with additional digestive enzymes helps alleviate some of the stress for digestive enzyme synthesis. With fatigue being an issue, taking an enzyme as soon as you begin to eat will help tax the body less and gain you more metabolic energy by improving the breakdown of your food.

Is there any downside to taking a digestive enzyme? If you take too many, you get hungry faster. In addition, they are safer to take than hydrochloric acid tablets, which when taken in excess can cause you to loose calcium and damage to your digestive track from the excessive acid. Furthermore, a digestive enzyme will help you break down carbohydrates, food additives, fats, fiber, and gluten by products, something that HCL will not do. HCL's primary function is to break down protein. This is why individuals taking HCL alone will often still suffer bloating, loose stool and/or constipation from ingesting carbohydrate and oils.

Another thing that you can do is to observe the size of your meals. Many individuals suffering from low energy have no appetite for most of the day. When they do eat, they either eat very little or eat one meal for the day. It's better to avoid taxing your digestive system with a large meal, especially because carbohydrate metabolism is often a challenge. Low cortisol tends to create low thyroid function. Both of which can slow the digestive process. Eating a small meal every 3 hours reduces the digestive stress on the body. Each meal should contain some protein. Eating every 3 hours helps you to have a more even blood sugar level throughout the entire day. This will help you to have improved energy and stamina and allow your adrenal glands to regain their strength when not being taxed by carbohydrate dominant meals.

What about supplements? If one were to consider over the counter supplementation, vitamin C (or orange juice provided your digestion can handle the acid), B12 (either methycobalamine or cyanocobalamine) and 5-tetra-hydrofolate (not folic acid) are your core three supplements that will help rebuild adrenal gland strength.

Should you also take an adrenal glandular supplement? I advise against it. What I have found consistently over the past decade in treating patients who are chronically ill, those that suffer immune disorders, food sensitivities, chronic candida and other fungal and dysbiotic gut issues, is that many have developed an immune sensitivity to cortisol. It is very similar to developing antibodies to one's thyroid hormones. However, having antibodies to cortisol is never routinely tested by allopathic medicine.

Developing an immune sensitivity to a hormone takes that hormone out of circulation for use by the body to the extent it is bound to an antibody. This depends upon the severity of the immune sensitivity. Your body is able to use some of the hormone, just a significantly lesser amount due to your body's immune reaction to it.

Taking a thyroid or adrenal glandular tissue supplement would then serve to prompt more of an immune reaction in individuals already suffering from inflammatory conditions and toxic retention. Many individuals who begin to take glandular supplements feel good initially. Then they start to feel worse the longer they take the glandular. Their body begins to mount an ever increasing reaction to the glandular tissue whether it is bovine, sheep or pig based. Your reaction to cortisol is more likely to occur when you have developed immune sensitivities based upon having had elevated cortisol or having taken exogenous cortisol over time.

Unless you know whether your immune system has become sensitized to your adrenal gland tissue (the cortex or medulla), or to cortisol itself or its precursor metabolites, taking a glandular supplement can backfire. Once your immune system has become sensitized to adrenal tissue or cortisol, inflammation triggers begin inhibiting its use. Thus, although you and your health care practitioner may be focused upon increasing your cortisol levels, if your immune system has become sensitized to cortisol, to the extent it is sensitive to cortisol, your overall level of inflammation will increase in direct proportion to the degree of immune sensitivity and overall level of inflammation present in the body.

A telltale sign that you might be developing an immune sensitivity to cortisol can be diminished benefit or even an adverse reaction when taking a cortisol promoting supplement or cortisol itself. It is often the case that with initial exposure to these supplements and/or cortisol you find your body reacts well and your energy improves. However, over time you can become reactive. When that occurs, the benefits diminish. This occurs more commonly in patients who have antibodies to thyroid hormone and/or thyroid tissue or suffer low grade chronic infections. Work with an experienced health care provider who can check for immune sensitivities to adrenal tissue and cortisol at the very minimum to determine if glandular supplements should be avoided.

If you have a high level of inflammation, have multiple chemical sensitivities, mold sensitivities, chronic infections and/or food sensitivities, it is best to avoid taking glandular supplements. Your immune system is at a higher state of alert. If it isn't already sensitized to adrenal cortex, adrenal medulla tissue or cortisol, then it can become so more easily than with someone with a less reactive immune system. Glandular products are protein based and 'foreign' in the sense that this protein comes from a non-human animal. When your body does not break down this glandular protein sufficiently, some of the complex protein molecules can remain in your circulation and turn on immune recognition, thus prompting the development of an immune sensitivity to that glandular. When your immune system is on a higher level of alert because of other infections or immune sensitivities, it's easier for your body to become sensitized to a smaller amount of circulating 'foreign' protein.

As far as exercise goes, no matter how exhausted or fatigued you are, walking is the best exercise. Make an effort to walk at least 20 minutes a day to get your blood moving and to move your body. Swing your arms freely and try to walk at a faster pace than you would walking to your car parked in the shopping center. Vary the pace and push yourself for 30 sec then resume a slower pace and repeat if you are just starting out. The goal initially is not target heart rate cardio but rather to move the body, move the blood circulation. When your blood circulation doesn't move, it's more difficult to eliminate the toxins from your body. Walking and moving also helps to bring oxygen to the tissues which help your body to alkalinize, improves cellular energy, and mental clarity! Pathogens hate oxygenated tissue which is one reason hyperbaric chambers are used to kill off infection from the "flesh eating bacteria" otherwise extremely resistant to most drugs.

If you are too ill to walk outside, walk around your home. Just try to move daily for starters. Recall the things you liked to do as a child activity wise for play. Was it tossing a basketball in a hoop, throwing a Frisbee, playing catch with a ball, tennis, some type of dance, riding a bike, or skating? You might be thinking right now you aren't a kid anymore and you certainly don't have the energy to act like one! However, I mention this to help you tie into the joy you felt with that particular activity because you can recreate smaller versions of those activities now. For example, if you liked to dance, you can search the internet YouTube channels for beginning lessons on a type of dance and just stand there and give it a 10 minute go. If you use to ride your bike everywhere you can ride a stationary bike with headphones to your favorite music and do it slow and steady.

The key is to enjoy moving your body. I have found the elliptical machine at the gym makes me feel like I'm cross country skiing. If you enjoy exploring and the outdoors you can find a nearby park and just walk its walkways. The change of scenery makes you forget yourself. The fresh air is uplifting to your mood and the movement helps you sleep better at night among other things. While trying to recover and escape your low energy trap I can't emphasize enough how important it is to find some joy in being, in using your body. Movement is the best way to be 'in' your body.

The positive movement/exercise experience will help send signals to the brain that your body can still do a lot and even helps signal it to prepare to do more! There is a biochemistry of exercise that involves increasing levels of enzyme synthesis and blood sugar metabolism that takes time to become efficient. Over time and repetition you will be able to do more and longer and get stronger. You will build stronger glands and an immune system while peeling off the layers that kept you stuck in your low energy trap. Therefore, do not have the mindset that you need to be able to go out and do a 30 minute high aerobic program to benefit. Start where you are at with your body. Just move it and rhythmically at a pace you can enjoy and your body will do the rest!

If you are more ambitious and go to a gym to work out, pace yourself. If you find that you are more fatigued or exhausted even two hours after your workout, you have done too much. You need to lessen the intensity of what you do. If you don't do that, you will wear your adrenal glands down even further!

Despite a popular myth, you cannot exercise your exhausted adrenals back into health. The wrong type or an excessive amount of physical activity only serves to stress the adrenal glands more. As your adrenal glands recover, you will see you are physically able to do more tasks with less fatigue afterward. You will be able to accomplish more during the day and even begin to enjoy physical activities that previously you wouldn't think of doing. This is another barometer your adrenal glands are getting stronger.

A caveat to consider is sometimes we think in order to recover from whatever has us in our low energy trap we have to run to the gym. We think we are just out of shape or need to get into shape after recovering from a condition. We throw ourselves into exercise in the hope it helps us to feel stronger and gain more energy every day. That is how it's supposed to work when there is no continuing lingering 'subclinical' infection. However, unless our cortisol levels are in normal range and not low or high and unless we are using our thyroid hormones when our lab values show that they are in normal range, our endurance will be impacted by vigorous aerobic exercise. In fact, we can even weaken our adrenal and thyroid glands by taxing them with too aggressive exercise programs.

Moderation is the key and the best way to determine if we are moderating our exercise program is to monitor our fatigue a couple of hours after exercise. As our strength and endurance improves so will the post work out fatigue as long as we haven't overdone. You might be able to walk 20 minutes on a treadmill and recover well but 40 minutes leaves you more tired the whole evening and lagging the next day. Back off and moderate your activity level so that you don't dip into your energy bank account. Seek the level of exercise that gives you more energy and mental clarity an hour or two afterward and does not leave you tired. This will help you operate best within your optimal metabolic and hormonal range.

Even more important is to address those issues mentioned in this book that might apply to you. As you do and begin to experience more energy, don't run out and do all the things you haven't been able to do in a day and exhaust yourself. If you do, you will weaken your glands. The key to remember is to not overtax your adrenals by doing too much in a day as you begin to find yourself having small bursts of energy. It never fails that I hear a patient say, "Oh I felt better one day and I decided to clean the entire garage, something I haven't been able to do in years, only to end up on the couch exhausted the next day or two." I tell the patient that as their adrenal glands become stronger they output a bit more cortisol. It's like a savings account in the bank. Don't go to town with it and bust your account. I explain. I advise them that they will begin to "see the clouds part on their energy" and will need to ration how they use that energy. Try not use it all up on all those things they haven't been able to do, otherwise, their "bank account" will be in the red again and they will feel exhausted and no better. Until the adrenal glands become strong enough to regularly output normal levels of cortisol, taxing them weakens and delays the process of recovery.

What Can You Do to Improve Excessive Cortisol Output?

During those times of day when your salivary cortisol biorhythm is excessive, there is much you can do to help reduce that output. Remember excessive cortisol causes excessive insulin output. Therefore, what you eat at the time of day when your cortisol is excessive can mean all the difference to your energy and whether you are gaining belly fat and weight in general.

The best thing to do if you have elevated cortisol anywhere in your saliva cortisol lab report is to note the time of day it is excessive. At that time of day you must avoid eating a large meal that includes carbohydrates. Rather, eat a small meal and leave out the carbohydrates. Eat a low carbohydrate meal, a small amount of potato, rice or root vegetables or none at all preferably at the time of day when your cortisol is high. And make sure to include protein at that meal.

You are more prone to insulin resistance when your cortisol is excessive. Therefore, you need to limit your carbohydrate intake at that time. This prevents fat storage and aggravation of insulin resistance resulting from eating too much carbohydrate for what your body is able to metabolize stemming from the imbalance in cortisol/insulin secretion.

In addition, it is essential to have even blood sugar throughout your day. This means no insulin spikes that come from eating too many carbohydrates for what your body can handle. This also means no blood sugar lows because of your insulin spike or because you skipped a meal and waited too many hours to eat between meals. Eating every 3 hours (9 a.m., noon, 3 p.m., 6 p.m., 9 p.m.) and making sure you have protein at each meal will help to reduce glandular and digestive stress (because of insulin output) to a more manageable level. Smaller and more frequent meals will reduce the insulin output. This will help to down-regulate the cell membranes to be less prone to ignoring insulin's signal thereby reducing insulin resistance. Eating every 3 hours, with protein at each meal, will help maintain better blood sugar levels throughout the day. You will gain better cellular nutrition and therefore better energy!

You also need to examine your lifestyle at the times of day when your cortisol output is high. What do I mean by this? Take a look at the time of day your cortisol is elevated and ask yourself "What am I doing at that time of day?" If you are working and you are under high stress at the office, and to deal with that pressure you are also drinking coffee/lattes etc. then you are biochemically stressing your adrenal glands to output excessive cortisol.

If the time of day when your cortisol is high finds you under family stress, you need to examine what is happening at home. Is it the time of day when you are trying to feed the family, help the kids with their homework and get them ready for the next day? Are you staying up late to finish a work project after the family has gone to bed? How you are coping at home with what life is asking you to do? Do you have enough help? Are you organized in your approach to getting things done.

Examine what you are doing and see if you can become more organized to do certain things a certain day and parcel the chores out rather than exhaust yourself trying to do it all at the time of day when your cortisol is elevated. Ask yourself "What is happening that is causing my body to register a stress response?" If you need to make changes to get your family to pitch in, speak up and delegate. You must stop trying to do "everything" especially at *that* time of day when your cortisol level is high. Pace yourself, and postpone those chores that pile up the stressors to a time of day when your cortisol is more normal and within a good range. If you are exercising when your cortisol is excessive, you must change the time you work out. If you cannot, you need to change to a relaxing form, such as walking or yoga to help ramp down the cortisol. You might not think that everything you are doing at that particular time is causing your adrenals to output excessive cortisol, but it is!

I have treated countless busy, fully employed yet exhausted individuals who knew they could not keep their pace going indefinitely. Some already had to take a leave of absence from work or cut their hours. Others were struggling to hold their full time jobs for lack of energy. One patient of mine had high cortisol output at the dinner hour. I asked her what she was doing at that time and she said "the normal family stuff". Rushing home from work to pick up the kids, then make dinner and help the kids with homework while doing household chores. For her the sum total of what otherwise should be a normal family evening was taxing her and entombing her in a low energy trap. Soon she would be good for no one.

I asked her if she could put off some household chores to another time of day and on a weekend when her cortisol output was more normal. We also examined how much help she was getting from her spouse with the kids and she decided to sit down with her husband, show him her cortisol biorhythm and asked him to start to pick up the kids while she got home to cook. She also decided to cook larger meals with leftovers that could be made into different dishes the next day to lighten her cooking chores and to use a crock pot more so dinner would be ready when she got home. These small changes made her life less hectic and she was not only able to reduce her "perceived" stress of trying to "do it all", but was able to improve her adrenal biorhythm and enjoy her family more! Yes, day to day living and raising a family can be taxing but it is up to you to manage your stress and juggle your chores so as not to damage your adrenal glands!

I had another exhausted real estate executive with astronomical cortisol at noon. When I asked her what was going on at work that was causing her body to act like she was running from a freight train she confessed her boss held morning meetings and the stress from the pressure of those meetings literally "lit a fire" in her. She felt a fear/stress response while at work as a result. Besides giving her a supplement to help her detoxify her excessive cortisol, we worked on her perception of fear and stress with her boss to enable her to become more grounded and task oriented as opposed to fear focused. In a couple of months her cortisol dropped down to normal levels. Her racing heart and mind and exhausted yet racing feeling was replaced with a sense of accomplishment, empowerment and efficiency.

Another culprit of lifestyle that causes elevated cortisol output is overstimulation of the brain at night. Many people spend their entire evening on the computer, working, surfing the internet, playing internet games or chatting with family and friends, well into the wee hours of the night. They go to bed late and get less than six hours a night of sleep. You might think you are relaxed while you are sitting on the computer in the late evening, but this constant barrage of information your eyes take in from the computer keeps your brain in a constant state of stimulation. Brain stimulation perpetuates stimulatory brain chemistry which in turn stimulates the adrenal glands to keep secreting cortisol. What the brain should be doing is putting on the brakes and allowing the body to slow down and enter the sleep state.

Overstimulation of the brain from computers, TV, videogames, reading for prolonged periods of time and well into the evening hours prevents your body from biochemically and hormonally ramping down. Just because you close the book, turn off the TV or computer doesn't mean your body switches off like an appliance and you can then fall asleep.

In many cases, these individuals will also call themselves "night owls". They stay up too late, reducing the hours they can actually get rejuvenating sleep. Getting a minimum of six hours of sleep is essential and often not enough. Many health conditions stem from and are aggravated by sleeping six or fewer hours. Hypertension is just one of these conditions. A good rule of thumb is that you must be in bed by midnight and you must stop all mental stimulation at least one to two hours before bed. This means the computer shuts off at 10:00 p.m. if you are going to get up at 6:00 a.m.

An additional problem that aggravates excessive cortisol output which results from overstimulation of the brain at night, is the excessive output of norepinephrine and/or dopamine. In most cases I see excessive norepinephrine before bed. The person's brain is alert, very alert. Their body is tired but their brain won't shut off. Often, besides excessive cortisol, their brain has too much circulating norepinephrine. This can result from overstimulation of the brain but it can also result from the body's slow ability to detoxify one's norepinephrine, as with cortisol. I will discuss that shortly.

One cannot reduce excessive cortisol output if the lifestyle stressors (even when you do not perceive it as stress) are not addressed. Therefore, examine what you are routinely doing at that time of day when your cortisol is high and make some changes! Also examine if you are taking in stimulants. Tea, coffee and chocolate all contain caffeine. Cigarette smoking is a stimulant as is alcohol, even a glass of wine can throw off brain and hormone chemistry. You must not take stimulants at those times when your cortisol is high. To do so is to add tinder to an already roaring fire!

Exercise for those with elevated cortisol must also be adjusted. Try not to exercise at the time of day when your cortisol is high, as your first rule of thumb. If there are no normal cortisol values for when you can exercise that work with your lifestyle, then you have to change the type and intensity of your exercise.

If you have to work out when your cortisol values are high, you must not exercise strenuously at those times when your cortisol is high. To do so, makes your adrenal glands continue to work hard and your cortisol values will not come down. The type of exercise needed when cortisol is high is something that is calmer and stress relieving. Yoga, walking, tai chi, Pilates and stretching, a leisure bike ride, all provide rhythmic movement that helps to release stress from the body.

You should not jog, play competitive sports, racket ball, tennis, or weight lift when your cortisol is high. Remember that with elevated cortisol, you also have more inflammation because excessive cortisol increases inflammation. To perform strenuous exercise at the time of day when your body is biochemically under inflammatory chemical signals is very damaging and is contra productive to the benefits of the exercise you seek.

What supplements are best to take to lower high cortisol? Your health care practitioner will generally recommend phosphotidylserine. It comes in many different formulas by itself or trans-dermally. The key is to take it at the time of day when your cortisol is high. It will help your body break down and detoxify the excessive cortisol provided that your diet and lifestyle are not "fueling the fire".

An economical form of this fatty acid can be found in lecithin! Generally speaking, one serving contains over 3000 mg of phosphatidylcholine, the precursor molecule that your body uses to make phosphatidylserine. It is much cheaper than buying a supplement of phosphatidylserine. However, with patients that do not digest fats and fatty acids well, those with gallbladder problems or known sensitivities to soy and those with considerable digestive issues, lecithin will not be your best course of action and you will do better on a transdermal or pill supplement.

Get Retested!

With everything you are doing to increase or lower your cortisol values, it is essential to retest your salivary cortisol within 60 days, no more than 90 days after embarking on a treatment program to alter your cortisol levels. In this fashion, you get feedback as to the pace in which your adrenals are adjusting and improving, and you get feedback if you are now going to need to lower your dosage on any supplement or medication as your cortisol biorhythm comes into balance.

If you do not retest, thinking you will base your decision on how you are feeling from symptoms alone, you run the risk of elevating your cortisol levels or never getting them within normal range! Some supplements over time will actually overstimulate the adrenals. What was a low output of cortisol becomes excessive on the supplement. Remember elevated cortisol is often silent symptom wise unless prolonged and very elevated. Even then it takes testing to nail down elevated cortisol as the culprit. Therefore, taking a cortisol enhancing supplement without testing is bad! The only way to prevent elevation or suboptimal cortisol excretion is to monitor your levels with regular testing. In addition, as the adrenal glands improve in strength, you will no longer need your cortisol boosting supplements. This is why testing is an excellent monitor of your progress.

Once your cortisol biorhythm is within normal range, it may take a few months of continual low dose supplementation to maintain optimum cortisol levels. Most patients with low DHEA have to stay on a maintenance dose of DHEA to hold their normal DHEA levels. However, in the case of adrenal glands, once the source of chronic infection and viral loads are reduced, many patients are able to taper down on their adrenal gland supplementation over time provided they maintain good DHEA levels.

Bear in mind that you can strengthen your adrenal glands while you fight infection and optimize neurotransmitter and other hormonal functions. It may take longer depending upon how many systems are affected (thyroid, types of infections you are fighting). Therefore, keep these factors under consideration as you watch your adrenal glands respond to therapy and you gauge your progress with lab testing. You will gradually pull yourself out of your low energy trap!

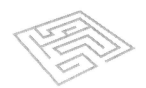

CHAPTER 8

WHEN
SUPPLEMENTS FAIL

A s I mentioned previously, chronic infection (dysbiosis, gingivitis, cavitations, Lyme disease, viral infections, chronic low grade bacterial infections, hidden parasitic, fungal, candida and yeast infection) all initially marshal the adrenal gland to output cortisol as part of its alarm signaling, immune stimulation response to attack. As the infection lingers and becomes chronic *and* as the patient begins to retain more toxins (from die off of pathogens, mal-absorption of medications and supplements and other factors too complicated for purposes of this book), these toxins will act as immune triggers. They will prompt the immune system into becoming sensitized to recognize cortisol as "foreign" due to the high levels now circulating in the body.

This is how you first develop an immune sensitivity to cortisol. It can occur during an acute illness from viral attack such as Epstein Bar. It can occur during your body's aggressive attempt to ward off infection from Lyme pathogens. Whatever prompts your immune system into a defense mode will increase your cortisol output. Over time, with increased cortisol circulating in your body, along with increased circulation of defensive immune cells, some of these cells will begin to view the circulating cortisol as 'bad' and develop an immune recognition to it. This reduces your body's ability to use cortisol and increases your inflammation further whenever cortisol secretion is increased.

As time progresses the adrenal glands fatigue. They struggle to output normal amounts of cortisol. Couple the fatigue of your adrenal glands with the fact your immune system has formed antibodies to cortisol, you now have less cortisol available for your cells to use. As a result, your cortisol levels drop. The downward cascade of chronic low cortisol levels along with all those accompanying symptoms begin to peak.

Since allopathic medicine does not now incorporate the concept of "functional medicine", it will not be concerned with optimizing low cortisol output or utilization and therefore will not look to monitor cortisol levels as a way of assessing optimization of adrenal function. By only looking for disease, blood tests will not discover this downward spiral of your "invisible" gland because standardized CBC panels do not test for serum cortisol. In addition, you now know that even if a serum cortisol test were run, it would not give you the data you need to know what your cortisol biorhythm is. Therefore, your true cortisol biorhythm and whether you have developed an immune sensitivity to your cortisol will totally escape 99% of allopathic medicine practitioners and another 99% of alternative medical (chiropractic, acupuncture, osteopathic, naturopathic, homeopathic) practitioners unless trained specifically for what to look for in treating adrenal fatigue and exhaustion. Of those trained to do salivary cortisol testing, 99% of those do not understand nor do they test for immune sensitivities to cortisol or the metabolites that result in its synthesis or degradation.

Therefore, if you begin to notice reactions to your adrenal supplements, you could be developing an immune sensitivity to an ingredient in the supplement or to a metabolite in the cortisol pathway or to cortisol itself. Most doctors/health care practitioners will simply put you on something different. If you have been told to switch to a different supplement or switch from a neutraceutical to an herb pill, herbal tincture, or homeopathic, in the hope that something will work better for you and you still react, then it's a red flag you have become sensitized to cortisol. Even when another product is found that helps, it often ends up not working the longer you take it because your immune system has become sensitized to cortisol or its metabolites. Unless you stop and reverse the immune sensitivity that causes the block in your body's ability to make, use and degrade cortisol, any supplement you take will in time give you problems or stop helping.

Another way immune sensitivities to cortisol commonly occur is by taking exogenous cortisol! When your body digests the exogenous cortisol pill inadequately, and your dysbiosis (largely undetected or untreated) prevents the full absorption of this exogenous cortisol through your digestive tract, what is left circulating in your lymphatic system and blood stream is undigested, un-metabolized and thus excessive cortisol. This circulating cortisol and its larger metabolites in effect become toxins that the immune system will begin to see as "foreign". The immune system will then become sensitized to "recognize" cortisol and bind it, taking that bound cortisol out of commission. How severe this is and how much cortisol your body reacts to varies depending upon the degree of inflammation in your body.

Many doctors do not realize nor do they watch for the sensitization to cortisol from taking exogenous cortisol. The same is true for exogenous thyroid hormone. Many patients first report their exogenous cortisol helped, but over time they didn't feel so well on it and took themselves off of it. The longer they took it the more they began to have reactions to it. That is a telltale sign that they had developed an immune sensitivity to the cortisol. Taking exogenous cortisol when you have other immune sensitivities and are in a higher state of inflammation is a sure fire way to develop a sensitivity to cortisol or any other exogenous hormone.

Immune Matrix is unique in the country in having a fast and efficient technology to test for immune sensitivities to cortisol on the spot. Our research has progressed to include testing for cortisol's key metabolites that are involved in its synthesis as well as its degradation. Based upon my research in over a dozen years, I have worked to identify those key metabolites that the immune system "recognizes" and the proprietary technology to identify positive signatures for immune interference.

At present, nothing exogenous (no supplement, herb, drug, or homeopathic) is available that can reverse immune sensitivities to cortisol. Some systems of treatment can be successful for a short time provided that the patient is not in a high level of inflammation and they are able to detoxify adequately to reduce the immune triggers. This is why it is so frustrating for most health care practitioners and so daunting for patients to see their energy getting worse while on a treatment protocol. It's even more daunting to see doctors doing everything but helping to rejuvenate adrenal glands.

Not knowing how to strengthen the adrenal glands, not knowing how to work with the immune system, to improve detoxification, and to remove those stressors that throw off one's cortisol biorhythm will leave you locked in your low energy trap because you will never rebuild your adrenal gland's strength. Treating the patient for these immune sensitivities by reversing the block the body has to using cortisol and allowing the adrenal glands to optimize cortisol production and detoxification is key.

The nuances of treating a gland that is largely ignored by allopathic medicine unless diseased are subtle. However, familiarity with cortisol biorhythm and its optimization can make a world of difference in allowing patients to regain their strength, vitality, metabolic function, immune stamina, blood sugar regulation, brain focus and stamina long before the organ reaches a disease state. Don't let your adrenal glands become the invisible glands. Take action to optimize your cortisol biorhythm and you will spring yourself out of your low energy trap!

You can improve your adrenal function and do it with natural supplements. You can normalize your cortisol function such that lifelong dependency on prescription cortisol is not necessary. Optimum cortisol function will improve your body's ability to use thyroid hormone. Optimal cortisol biorhythm will give you stamina and immune strength to break through chronic infections.

Treating adrenal insufficiency or excessive cortisol secretion is something that is not discussed in medical schools if it's not for the treatment of Cushing's or Addison's or anything shy of a disease classification. Optimizing cortisol function is ignored in allopathic medicine unless a category can be made up by Big Pharma to sell a drug outside a disease diagnosis or a fabricated disease diagnosis (i.e. as in the case of the little purple pill advertising a type of depression that does not exist in DMS-IV disease classification guidelines, a total marketing classification that somehow slipped by the FDA). But that is another story for another book. So the fact a drug doesn't exist for the treatment of low or high cortisol doesn't mean it's not a problem, or that it's not a disease. You must take your biological markers into your own hands. Seek the best treatment and supplementation protocol that gets you out of your low energy trap. Don't wait to be told you have a disease and don't be fooled into complacency by the well-meaning ignorance of some health care professionals who try to tell you that you are fine when you don't feel fine.

CHAPTER 9

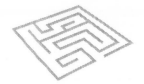

THE LIMITATIONS OF ALLOPATHIC MEDICINE

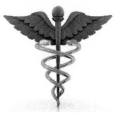

Time and again patients ask me "Why didn't my doctor (allopathic) tell me this?" I have to explain that in part it's not the fault of your allopathic doctor if you understand the system that he/she operates in.

What options does allopathic medicine (Western medicine) offer someone in a low energy trap? When you pass through the hospital/clinic doors of your local allopathic hospital or treatment center, what road are you traveling? Health care in the United States is dominated by allopathic medicine for good and not so good reasons depending upon the condition. Yet other parts of the world have other dominate systems (Ayurveda, Chinese Medicine, Homeopathy, and Osteopathy to name a few). When you go to your "Western" doctor you have plugged yourself into the allopathic medical model and the allopathic tool box of fixes. You need to know where you are (the allopathic model) and what road it takes you to see if it will lead you to where you want to go.

If you want non-drug solutions, natural options and choices, then you can't bemoan your traditional Western medical doctor's disease focus, prescription drug approach. If he or she fails to advise you that a certain supplement or herb can lower your cholesterol, blood pressure and/or improve your blood sugar as a first option over being given a prescription drug, remember that their training is first drug based. Furthermore, depending upon the institution the doctor is employed with, prescription drugs may be his or her only tool in the bag. Most doctors working for hospitals and large medical centers are institutionally prohibited as a matter of economic policy from recommending anything but a prescription drug and only certain low cost drugs at that!

Neither can you trust your allopathic doctor's opinion about other systems of medicine unless they have personally studied the system themselves. Too many people voice ignorant opinions about subjects they never took the time to study. For me to say quantum physics is bunk is entirely unprofessional and idiotic if I have never studied quantum physics. That goes for any alternative system of medicine. Each system has its limitations including allopathic medicine, yet those limitations do not necessarily make that entire system of medicine invalid. If so, allopathic medicine would have been invalid years ago for its myriad failures in surgeries, medical theories of bleeding with leeches to cure illnesses to shock therapy to heal every suspected psychiatric condition. The misuse, improper use or overuse of a modality of treatment is not sufficient to invalidate an entire system of medicine. Therefore, keep your perspective and objectiveness when discussing the opinions and uneducated biases of those that seek to be an authority in one field but clearly are not one in another!

Why do we allow someone with expertise in one field carte blanche to voice an opinion in a field and in an area they never studied, or didn't study enough of? Remind your health care provider that unless they have studied the subject of what they are espousing sufficiently more than a weekend continuing education seminar's worth, they are making a very unprofessional statement.

Let me give you an example of a doctor I knew who took a weekend acupuncture course designed for doctors so that they themselves could do acupuncture on patients and therefore not have to hire a fully trained acupuncturist or refer their patients out. In California and most states that I am aware of, one must have at least three years of training before one qualifies to sit for the State Board Exam to become a Licensed Acupuncturist.

This doctor takes a weekend course and the following week inserts acupuncture needles in a patient's knee. When the patient did not improve, he concluded that acupuncture didn't work. We were having a phone call about his experience and I began to ask him questions when he told me did acupuncture on his patients knee and it didn't work. I asked him if he used electro-acupuncture, or just needles and if so, how often did he stimulate the needles and how. I asked him what point combinations did he use. How long was the treatment he gave the patient? Combinations he asked? Stimulation? There are point combinations he said? What is electro acupuncture? I asked him if he used any 'master points'? What are 'master points' he replied. What was your Chinese medical diagnosis for his knee I asked? Did you use 5 element theory or some other theory?

He was totally stunned and befuddled and realizing that there was more to acupuncture than poking an acupuncture needle around a patient's knee. He replied that he really therefore didn't understand how to apply the needles aside from knowing what points were available to be used. He confessed that he assumed if he just put the needles around where the knee was in the acupuncture points he learned from his weekend seminar they would help the patient.

I explained that as an allopathic doctor, just because you can stick a needle in someone, sure you can learn to properly insert an acupuncture needle in a patient, but you have to do the proper Chinese medical diagnosis. Without the proper diagnosis you don't know what point combinations to apply. The diagnosis dictates the acupuncture point combinations to use depending upon what you are trying to accomplish. Are you trying to tonify and fortify the tendon or reduce inflammation or increase circulation or a combination thereof. Each acupuncture point will do different things. The rehabilitation of the knee, reduction in inflammation, or strengthening of a ligament all require different approaches the same with allopathic medicine or physical therapy. I told him if he wanted to be effective he needed to study more, way more. I told him that his weekend class gave him but an intro into what acupuncture was but in no manner can any weekend course on any system of medicine cover all its uses. He thanked me and promptly referred the patient to an acupuncturist.

Make sure you seek expert opinions from people who are experts in that particular field of study. Ask them if they have formally studied herbs, chiropractic, homeopathy, acupuncture, Chinese medicine, Aruveda, neutraceuticals, neutrigenomics etc. and for how long. Ask them about their certifications before asking them a question pertaining to that particular science. You don't ask your plumber about electrical issues do you? Even though both work on houses, the training is entirely different.

This is why I'm taking great pains to state what some say is obvious but many of us don't realize, that the training, traditions, and tools provided your M.D. are limited to surgery, prescription drugs and talk therapy. Time and time again I find myself explaining to patients frustrated with allopathic medicine that their doctors never received training in the benefits of specific neutraceutical brain supplements, the use of specific neutraceuticals such as CoQ10, the benefits of a qEEG not to mention what it even is or how to optimize vitamin D levels, or identify detoxification issues. I explain to them that all these things and more fall outside "disease" treatment parameters.

This is why I say to YOU, "Know the road you are on so that you can determine if it will lead you to the health outcomes you seek". Alternative, integrative and functional health care practitioners have a responsibility to educate their patients about the field of healthcare they are in and help the patient to have the proper prospective about the benefits and limits of different types of medicine. Gone should be the days when one system is trashed entirely out of competitive strife when another treatment modality is more appropriate for a particular issue. Optimizing our strengths and acknowledging our limitations is for the good of the patient, as is patient education so that they can make the best choice for their recovery. Isn't that is what matters in the end, recovery?

This book is designed to help you see the big picture about those little discussed issues that keep you locked in your low energy trap and to help you systematically isolate and address each issue. It is designed to prevent you from succumbing to the prevailing and inevitable resignation that you will have to adjust to living a low energy lifestyle because your doctors have run out of answers. Understanding the limits and pitfalls in any system of medicine will help you to optimize your options with renewed focus and treatment strategies!

Understanding that allopathic medicine is the dominant medical system in this country with the most insurance support will also help you gain perspective. It is why most individuals choose the allopathic route because it is most easily covered by insurance. However, it funnels you into the "disease" model. It is another reason for teeth gnashing by so many patients I see, frustrated why the things I mention in this book were not addressed with their insurance covered plans. I remind them insurance coverage is largely focused on disease. I cannot therefore emphasize enough how important it is for you to abate your frustrations in obtaining answers by understanding the focus as well as the tools used in each system of medicine in order to determine if that system offers you what you now need to escape your low energy trap.

Being your own best detective to unearth the causes for your chronic fatigue will ensure your escape. You can do more to improve your health by seeking those roads that "optimize" your health. Even with a disease diagnosis you can optimize your health! Those roads are there to lead you to the answers you need to peel away the layers of what keeps you locked in your low energy trap. I passionately encourage you to learn, discern, and continue to be your own detective!

ALLOPATHIC MYOPIA

When I see many a patient of mine frustrated that their doctor didn't unveil the causes that keep them in their low energy trap and exclaim 'Why?, I remind them their frustration comes from failing to see and accept things the way they are. Sometimes you can be a vehicle for change but first one must deal with the frustration of moving that wheel ever so slowly and with great effort. This only happens with knowledge and education. First you have to see allopathic medicine's strengths and weaknesses. Then, don't limit yourself based upon the limits of allopathic medicine's narrow view of having a disease only focus or its "limited" tool box of treatments for the treatment of diseases when what is wrong with you may substantially go beyond any disease diagnosis.

Successful treatment options are available to improve your health beyond the scope of prescription drugs, talk therapy or surgery. It is said that "medicine is an art", and all forms of medicine (osteopathic, acupuncture, Chinese Medicine, Ayurveda, chiropractic, homeopathy, naturopathy) learn through trial and error (on our patients with trial and observation). It's the nature of all medical systems in general to be slow to change and evolve, as only time proves trial and error applications through the treatment of hundreds if not thousands of patients. That being said, allopathic medicine in the United States is even slower to broaden its focus and its tools from that of just disease based focus and treatment as compared to other systems of medicine and other countries.

Did you know there are hospitals in Europe using just essential oils and hospitals in China that use acupuncture instead of anesthesia for surgery, all quite successfully?! As an acupuncturist, I have induced and helped a mother stay in labor with ear acupuncture, preventing the need for labor inducing drugs, so that the mother could be drug free for delivery. It wasn't difficult to do and saved the hospital money. So why aren't more such applications routinely done?

Why is the public not told of their "alternative" options? Are alternative options not offered because they displace the use of a more profit inducing drug and thus bring in higher revenue for the hospital? Why is it up to you to be your own detective and demand natural, safer options? Why are you being forced to pay out of pocket for those natural options? These natural options do bring cures. Their use helps to avoid more costly side effects from prescription drugs that create dependency and often come with no hope of cure. So why aren't more of these beneficial options covered by insurance?

VICTIM MENTALITY

Disease is a compelling reason to focus one's resources for "a cure". From Girolamo Fracastoro's fifteenth century postulation that diseases were contracted by 'seed-like' entities transmitting infection via contact, to the father of microbiology, Anton van Leeuwenhoek's observation of microbes and disease transmitting vectors, allopathic medicine has and continues to embrace the "germ theory". The Black Death and Yellow Fever epidemics certainly fueled the need to get to the bottom of why entire villages perished.

Germ theory also fuels the prevailing attitude that we are still victims of infection and disease. Fear of new and emerging viruses that could plague us foster the feverish development of every new vaccine possible to flood the market and be given to younger and younger individuals for fear of succumbing to some feared or dire condition.

It is true germs are vectors for disease. However, research in the last few years now acknowledges and directly attributes our daily habits known as 'lifestyle' as significantly contributing to many life-shortening diseases. They include but are not limited to heart disease, stroke and diabetes. The National Center for Health Statistics, National Office of Vital Statistics as far back as 1900 reported that degenerative diseases account for at least 60 percent of all deaths in the United States. (Technical Notes NVSR, volume 48, page 11) Degenerative disease are conditions such as Alzheimer's disease, Parkinson's Disease, multiple sclerosis, atherosclerosis, cancer, diabetes, heart disease, rheumatoid arthritis, osteoarthritis and osteoporosis as well as broader named conditions such as irritable bowel and inflammatory bowel disease to name a few.

Furthermore, from what we now know about nutrition, certain lifestyle dietary choices contribute to nutritional imbalances. These imbalances in nutritional chemistry contribute to toxic retention, detoxification inefficiency, and acid terrain all of which foster the growth of pathogens and inhibit enzyme and hormone function. Therefore, your lifestyle habits can be the lock that keeps you in your low energy trap!

Many diseases are now being attributed to the result of bad lifestyle choices or choices that over time prevent the optimization of your hormones, your metabolism and digestion. Science is now also revealing how these choices trigger our weakest genetic tendencies. We can no longer say we are a victim of our genes! Lifestyle practices, day in and day out over the span of years leads us down a slippery slope toward suboptimal biochemistry, function and therefore disease. Only now is science and medicine beginning to acknowledge that as much as 80% of all disease can be prevented and even reversed when one changes daily habits of living. If we are victims, it is of ignorance. Science and medicine owes it to the public to educate, educate, educate.

Isn't it time we take what we know to emphasize and change our focus to prevent what is preventable? What is at stake? The loss of money from all those prescription medications we would not have to take for the next 10, 20 or 30 years if we never came down with hypertension, osteoporosis, high cholesterol or diabetes! There are billions of dollars at stake to keep us in the prescription drug pool!

Sad to say, economics of allopathic medicine do affect your health! There is no financial incentive to stay healthy and be healthy when Big Pharma takes it to the bank supplying the disease industry and your doctor with incentives to prescribe a certain number of pills or choose a more expensive drug over another. Drug reps watch what drug and amount your doctor prescribes. Their visits to your doctor are geared to influence and limit their choice in how they treat disease toward improving profitability for the drug manufacturing industry.

Furthermore, many hospitals, in an effort to control cost, do not allow their doctors to prescribe the "latest" and therefore most effective antibiotics. Many doctors complain about being corralled into prescribing from an "approved list of drugs", now less effective because of newer and costlier drugs that reduce the bottom line profits of hospitals. The purpose is cost control and not to optimize your health!

These practices go on behind your back daily. Doctors in private practice have more free rein to choose the latest antibiotic for example, than those working in membership hospitals. They have the least freedom. Which one are you going to get the best "drug" care from?

We are also led by the collective and historical attitudes of allopathic medicine that "disease is the inevitable ravage of getting older", and that "we are the inevitable victims of our genes". Don't believe it! Education and empowerment of the people is the best way to ensure our right to prevention and our right to seek natural non-pharmaceutical medical options. Taking early action nearly guarantees you won't have to go down that road.

NO TIME

Another reason your allopathic doctor might not have told you a number of helpful things is they have little time when they see a patient. Furthermore, in speaking to my doctor colleagues, time and again I notice they have an assumption that it's *too time consuming* to educate their patients on what and how they can prevent and/or reverse the progression of their symptoms that lead to disease. If they have five minutes with you they are right!

I talk to allopathic doctors all the time who have given up "trying" to educate their patients about what they can do. They have taken on the belief (falsely) their patients just want their prescription pad filled out, that their patients don't want to take responsibility to change what they are doing that could be causing, contributing or exasperating their condition. With some patients this is true but if you are reading this, you are not one of them!

When it's an uphill battle to convince a doctor to keep trying to educate their patients about prevention and lifestyle, you can see why the public is left in the dark about their true options. If options are not even broached, how is a patient to find out there is more to investigate? Profit's time constraints further limit your allopathic doctor's time and options for your health care.

Yes it's true that many people don't want to change their diet, or daily habits. They don't want to admit they are largely to blame for their state of ill health after years of bad choices made daily. These individuals are more than happy to take their prescription insulin, cholesterol and hypertension pills and change very little if nothing in their diet or lifestyle. These individuals lie to themselves that they are a victim of their genes. They make excuses pointing to family members that share their condition so that they really don't have to take responsibility to do the hard work it takes to reverse and improve their odds of not succumbing to the fate of their genes! They don't want to see and learn how what they eat daily contributes and causes their fatigue or other medical conditions because it means they will have to change, or worse yet stop the mindless eating and drinking of whatever they want.

In many cases it's too late to reverse a condition when they find out they have developed cancer or diabetes for example, but not always. In many cases, efforts to change one's lifestyle do improve symptoms, reverse conditions and reduce or eliminate one's need for prescription drugs.

On the other hand, many a doctor is to blame for leading such individuals into a false sense of security their disease is under control "so long as" they stay on their meds. Patients too are told they are stuck with their condition because they are getting "older" or it "runs in the family". These are truly outdated belief systems modern medicine is proving wrong every day! What do you want to believe? Do you believe your disease diagnosis is solely to blame for keeping you in your low energy trap and that it cannot improve any further? Do you truly believe there are no answers out there that can nudge you closer to escaping your low energy trap? What you believe will dictate what options you think could be available to improve your health.

If you are shocked to hear that age does not lead to inevitable disease, you need to keep reading about lifestyle, epigenetics, and nutrition. All three affect your genes to either help heal and repair the body or keep you stuck in your low energy trap! The World Health Organization held a podcast interview with Dr. Tim Armstrong from the WHO Department of Chronic Diseases and Health Promotion back in January 9, 2009, episode 56. In his interview, he spoke of how healthy lifestyle makes a significant difference. He said over four years ago the evidence is "now overwhelming" that lifestyle changes in diet and activity improve the health of entire communities! Have you seen significant changes in our health care despite this "overwhelming" evidence? No! I hate to suggest profit is not found in prevention or shortening disease outcomes but economics often rules health care policy.

Dr. Armstrong in his wisdom further spoke of a research project called "A Healthy Heart" were mass media was used to educate people about healthy nutrition, food labels, and the introduction of half portions in fast food restaurants as well as using healthy snacks in school coupled with more physical activity. It was a community focus. The local government announced automobile free days and built bicycle lanes! Smoking was banned in the workplace. Initially only 14% of the participants were deemed to have a healthy diet and after four years that increased to 30%.

Dr. Armstrong emphasized that 60% of all deaths are from non-communicable diseases (diseases that are not caused by pathogens) such as many cancers, heart disease, and diabetes. That number sadly has continued to grow to where it is now up to 80% of all chronic illness can be attributed to lifestyle! Dr. Armstrong further stated that all these diseases have common risk factors traced to lifestyle factors such as tobacco use, inappropriate diets, and physical inactivity.

Dr. Armstrong's data supported his findings to show that a simple 30 minutes a day of moderate physical activity reduces one's risk of heart attack by 50%. Increasing fruit and vegetable consumption can reduce the incidence of colon cancer by 50%. We need to continue to heed his wise counsel.

The WHO (World Health Organization) is trying to encourage governments around the world to create policies and infrastructure to support an environment that enables people to make better choices and live a healthier disease-free life as a result. The benefits to society as a whole in reducing health care costs make it a win-win situation.

The change in focus to disease prevention is only now getting more attention. The first global ministerial conference on healthy lifestyles and non-communicable disease control was held in Moscow in April 2011. International efforts can help put pressure on lagging governments, America is one. Dr. Armstrong mentioned in his 2009 interview that Iran was "an excellent example…(whose) principles can be applied to other …countries." In 2000, the WHO ranked America 38th in the world in health. We were not top 10 and have dropped further down the list in ranking, being the obese fast food nation of "prosperity" that we are.

HOW DOES A DISEASE ONLY FOCUS IMPACT YOUR TREATMENT OPTIONS & YOUR HOPE TO INCREASE YOUR ENERGY?

With ongoing efforts emphasizing the prevention of disease, the limiting factor in allopathic medicine's disease only focus must give way to a broader perspective that legitimizes early action, lifestyle changes and non-drug interventions to prevent disease. Its historical system of looking at the body from the lens of disease systems and their treatment will do nothing to prevent or optimize health.

One can be unhealthy and not have a disease. Based upon the focus of treating disease therefore, what most people do not realize is the laboratory tests your allopathic doctor has you take are geared to detect and diagnose disease states. They are not focused on optimizing your health, neither are they trained or prepared to counsel or treat you to prevent the development of a preventable condition or disease! This is why someone can see their doctor complaining of diabetic symptoms (thirst, frequent urination, among other things) and be told they are not diabetic because their lab values have not crossed the threshold to classify them as diabetic. But do you wake up one day suddenly diabetic? No! Allopathic medicine has the main focus of treating disease and unless and until your labs say you are diabetic, you will be told you don't have diabetes. That doesn't mean you are healthy! It also speaks of no preventative intervention by your doctor to empower you to change the course and progression of your symptoms to prevent you from getting diabetes. This is why the prevailing attitude of many a patient is that they fell victim to their disease, having no idea that years prior they could have altered the progression toward that diagnosis.

Unfortunately, this is how allopathic medicine proceeds for many conditions including low thyroid function, doing nothing until you one day suddenly test positive for a disease. Many an individual sits exhausted before their doctor and is told that their thyroid values are "fine". I ask many a patient "What does being told you are "fine" by your allopathic doctor mean?" The patient can't tell me. I tell them that in most likelihood their doctor has based that "fine" conclusion upon normal TSH and T3 (total T3) values.

When I insist on checking their labs, in most cases that doctor/hospital never tested for free T3, the actual amount of thyroid hormone "free" and not bound to proteins and therefore available for cells to use! When we test for free T3 we often see low values, explaining in part their fatigue. It means that even though they have sufficient quantities of thyroid hormone circulating in their bloodstream, the "free" and unbound amount of thyroid is too low to feed their cells. That also assumes that there is sufficient iodine attached to their cell receptor sites to allow the free thyroid hormone to enter the cell.

CAUSES ARE IGNORED

Another limitation in allopathic medicine is with its focus on treating the "symptoms" of disease. The cause is overlooked in the process of making the patient feel better. Many a doctor has told me their patients "don't care why, they just want a prescription". That may be true for those patients that seek relief in a pill. However, for those "holistic" patients, who prefer never to take over the counter or prescription drugs, they want to prevent and get to the root of a condition. They take the view of treating symptoms as ignoring the cause and therefore the eventual cure.

An example is the chronic use of antibiotics to treat vasculitis, an infection in the veins. The patients we have seen have all been told by their allopathic doctors that their only hope was to stay on antibiotics indefinitely. When we asked them what bacterial strains were causing their flare ups they did not know. Their records revealed little in the way of any lab findings performed to determine which species of pathogen their antibiotic prescription was attempting to eradicate.

Patients at Immune Matrix are tested to determine which bacterial strains their immune system tests weak to fighting. That is used as a red flag in determining possible chronic strains of infection. When the patient is treated to boost immune recognition for those strains they previously tested weak to fighting, their ability to find and eradicate the pathogen is enhanced. This makes their taking an antibiotic or anti-microbial tincture or remedy much more effective. Patients are then able to stop the cycle of recurrent infection. At first the flare ups are less severe. Then the flare ups are less frequent. Soon they rarely if ever have a flare up. This is an example of how finding the cause for a problem leads to the termination of the problem.

Another example is migraine. Many a patient is given a very strong prescription to combat the debilitating symptoms of migraine. Does it allow the patient to function better, or have migraines less frequently? No, it merely helps the patient to "ride out" the migraine episode with less agony. There is no attempt to identify the migraine trigger(s). Many incorrect assumptions are made as to what those triggers might be when advising migraine patients.

Patients at Immune Matrix are tested with a proprietary computerized technology to determine what those migraine triggers are. The triggers are often due to immune sensitivities to one's hormones, mineral salts, sugars, preservatives and food additives, and can be originating from old head traumas that alter one's electrical brain waves.

Migraines that stem from old head traumas originate in a part of the brain that can be identified by a qEEG (qualitative EEG) allowing for effective treatment with neurofeedback. When the triggering cause can be identified, the frequency, duration and severity of the migraine can be substantially reduced and in most cases eliminated. If all you take is a strong prescription pain pill, you have no hope of improvement or cure! Trying to recovery from recurrent migraine attacks will keep you in your low energy trap!

Most inflammatory diseases can be eliminated when the triggers are identified and addressed. Unfortunately, allopathic medicine seeks to suppress the immune reaction to quiet the symptoms. However, suppression of the immune system has its consequences and does not always work in the long run to prevent symptoms. Conditions falling into this category are asthma, irritable bowel, acid reflux, food allergies/sensitivities, environmental and chemical sensitivities, endometriosis, headache, migraine, PMS, ADD, OCD, autism, Crohn's disease, Hashimoto's thyroiditis, Wilson's syndrome, insomnia, anxiety disorders, many forms of depression, Lyme disease, vasculitis, lupus, chronic fatigue, arthritis, osteoporosis, and eczema to name a few.

Any and all these conditions contribute to various degrees of fatigue and cyclical low energy. These conditions affect and weaken the glands and lead to low hormone function in these glands. That is why to improve one's energy, the causes for chronic inflammation have to be addressed. One must look at causative triggers to change the course and progression of a condition.

WHAT CAN YOU DO?

As you are now beginning to see, chronic low energy has many culprits and these culprits go largely unidentified in a "disease focused" medical system. With exception to the most innovative and astute medical practitioners, your treatment options for low energy are limited when the lens or toolbox of your doctor is limited. Understanding how you could have slipped through the cracks with allopathic medicine is crucial for knowing that there are other medical causes that impact your optimizing nutritional absorption, brain chemistry, adrenal function, and identifying hidden sources for low grade infection that sap your immune system and thus your energy.

What can you do? Keep learning. Take the information given in this book and use it like a detective to isolate and eliminate all the causes for your low energy. Take the information given herein and discuss it with your doctor to ensure the proper labs are requested. You can also contact Immune Matrix through our blog www.chronicfatigueandnutrition.com to have us consult with your doctors to assist you in determining what tests should be done and why. We regularly work as a team with other doctors to troubleshoot and oversee treatment protocol effectiveness.

Finally, examine lifestyle factors that might be impacting your energy and make systematic changes. Remember that these changes may individually not cause a huge symptom reversal. However, just like peeling the layers off an onion, collectively and consistently, when enough is done, you will spring out of your low energy trap and reach new levels of vitality and energy. Remember too metabolism takes time to change just as going to the gym one day or one week doesn't turn you into a fitness model. It takes consistency to see sustained increments of improvement.

Do not become discouraged when you don't see the expected improvements in your energy. Take that as a sign that you either have not discovered all the factors keeping you in your low energy trap or are missing a crucial application. This doesn't mean you abandon what you are currently doing, as this could be what is keeping you from feeling worse! Stay the course and continue to seek answers and over time you will bring your health to new plateaus.

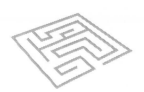

Chapter 10
ASK IMMUNE MATRIX

I f you would like a phone consult or find out how you can receive a comprehensive metabolic/immune evaluation, please call 888-519-5755 to find the clinic nearest you. For further articles by Anna Manayan, and to contact her via email for consultations, speaking engagements or lectures, send your inquiries to the blog: www.chronicfatigueandnutrition.com

IS THIS YOU?

Often when we suffer from low energy, we may know we have other medical conditions that contribute to keeping us in our low energy trap. The art and science of medicine is to unravel the interconnections of how an imbalance in one system can throw of the optimum performance of another system, or worse, lead to the development of other conditions in a downward cascade. Allopathic medicine's disease focus targets and isolates disease as part of its mode of operation and treatment. Integrative, alternative and functional medicine strives to look at each system and its collective effect in optimizing or throwing off the balance of other systems. Therefore, it often catches the downward spiral leading to the development of other conditions before they become separate entities requiring drug management.

Read the testimonials to help you begin to see how one condition sets up a person to develop another condition that when addressed resolves multiple symptoms and conditions. Support and balance is recovered to those systems that would otherwise slowly spiral downward into more entrenched conditions and fan out to begin new conditions.

Testimonial #1:

My daughter had recurrent stomach pains that caused her to eventually be on a severely restricted diet. She began to miss school more frequently because of her tummy disturbances for lack of a better word. She was tired often, listless and cranky. Her pediatrician had no explanation for the cause for her symptoms but decided to give her Zantac, which did nothing. After receiving an evaluation by Immune Matrix we discovered to our surprise extensive food sensitivities that affected her ability to break down protein, oils and carbohydrates. We discovered she had a severe overgrowth of bad flora in her digestive system as well as candida. I had no idea! After two months of treatment her stomach pains are gone and her appetite is returning as well as her sunny playful disposition.

Testimonial #2

My six week old baby cried so much something wasn't right. When she did eat her tummy would bloat. Then suddenly she began to refuse my breast milk and I was so worried she wouldn't thrive. She cried all the time and was becoming more listless in between her crying bouts. She stopped having bowel movements and she would scream for hours. The doctors wanted to surgically remove a part of her colon saying she had a fistula. Desperate to avoid surgery, we took her to Immune Matrix and found a host of food sensitivities. Needless to say she healed without the need for surgery and was able to continue breastfeeding thanks to their computerized assessment and non-invasive treatment program. She is now the spunky baby she should be, eating, pooping and thriving! Why didn't my pediatrician catch the causes?

Testimonial #3

After a severe attack of what appeared to be the flu, my child suffered a seizure. The pediatrician wanted to start anti-seizure meds immediately. We wanted to avoid having to put our child on prescription medication knowing it could go on indefinitely. Our child's demeanor had changed. There was less energy for play, difficulties focusing and we feared another seizure. So we sought an evaluation with Immune Matrix.

We found that our child had a weakened immune system to specific pathogens and had developed some food sensitivities. After undergoing their treatment program, we saw the frequency and severity of our child's seizure diminish until a year later there are no seizures. A QEEG at the time and now show that our child's brain has healed from the seizure site. Had we gone the allopathic seizure med route, our child would still be on drugs and probably still have the seizure focus that causes the seizures. Our child's energy and mental focus is back to normal and even our child's pediatrician is amazed that no seizure medications are needed. Why aren't more doctors learning this method of diagnosis and treatment?

Testimonial #4

I'm over 80 years old and have suffered eczema most my life. At the time I was told to get evaluated at Immune Matrix my rashes were in bad shape. They were red, swollen and oozing. I was skeptical because I've had eczema nearly all my life! However, I discovered what foods were causing it. I was skeptical it was nearly that simple, but I decided to give their advice a try. I'd been eating these foods all my life and not one doctor told them they contributed or aggravated my eczema! I learned how to cleanse my body property from the inside out. My skin healed for the first time in my life and I am eczema free. My bowel movements are no longer an issue. I thought I'd have to live with my bowel issues too. I thought that was just me. Now I have more energy than my children in their 50s!

Testimonial #5

Were it not for the testing and treatment program of Immune Matrix to discover that I had developed an immune sensitivity to progesterone, I would not have been able to complete my in-vitro fertilization program. I started to suffer severe side effects from the hormone injections. Headache, fatigue and rashes were turning my life upside down. Their de-sensitization program allowed me to stay on target with my IVF program and now I have a healthy happy baby!

Testimonial #6

When I came to Immune Matrix I had peculiar skin outbreak on the palms of my hands and feet. No M.D. was able to discern its cause despite extensive lab testing. After my initial evaluation with Immune Matrix I discovered I had food sensitivities to gluten, gliadin, and glutenin. My doctors told me I didn't test positive to Celiac or Crohn's and so I was told I could eat gluten. Well they were dead wrong! The treatment program at Immune Matrix was different to say the least, but I did the detoxification and treatments. It has helped me eliminate that annoying rash and I have lost weight as a result of their detoxification/purification/treatment program. I received other unexpected benefits as well. More energy, elimination of my bloating, improved digestion, sleep and brain function are my bonuses!

Testimonial #7

As a chronic insomniac for over 10 years, I was skeptical that I could get off my sleep meds and ever feel good when I woke up in the morning. However, after evaluation by Immune Matrix I discovered I had developed immune sensitivities to some of my neurotransmitters that affect mood and sleep. As I progressed in my treatment program I was able to be weaned off my sleep meds. My energy improved. The quality of my sleep improved, as did my mood. Had I not taken the chance to get evaluated I would still be on sleep meds and probably more drugs for depression. No one would have guessed or been able to determine that I had developed an immune sensitivity to some of my neurotransmitters!

Testimonial #8

Suffering from chronic brain fog, declining mental focus, fatigue, and loosing hope on life, I was urged by friends to go to Immune Matrix. They discovered that I had a high level of heavy metal retention and my liver was stressed by toxic retention even though my liver blood panels looked good according to my traditional M.D.. After undergoing Immune Matrix's detoxification program and being guided on how to safely eliminate my stored heavy metals, my brain clarity began to come back like a fog that lifted. I could focus longer and my energy began to return. I thought it was all just due to aging and faster than I wanted to. I am astounded how this issue of heavy metal toxicity can have such a huge impact on one's health. It's turned around my life and given me more energy, more life to my years!

Testimonial #9

I had to drop out of school for health reasons. My energy was so low I spent my days on the couch after getting up in the afternoon! My mom took me for evaluation by Immune Matrix and it was discovered that I had Rocky Mountain Spotted Fever, Epstein Bar and Lyme disease. That is a lot of bad news! What was worse was finding out how run down my adrenal glands had become and as a result my sugar metabolism and my immune system was not efficient in fighting. All I knew is that I was tired and ached all the time. After undergoing treatment, they were able to boost my cortisol and my body's ability to fight these pathogens. In time I began to feel stronger and stronger until I was able to return to high school. I did even better than that because I thought I'd never return to school. I graduated, went on a trip out of the country with no lapses in energy and am now a college student! Thank you for turning my life around!

Testimonial #10

I've seen many doctors for year round chronic sinus infections. I was constantly on antibiotics and my digestion was suffering more and more. My energy lagged, my head felt so foggy. I had pressure in my head all the time. I saw no end to this antibiotic routine the doctors had me on. I came for evaluation and Immune Matrix put me on their detoxification and treatment program. I discovered many foods I had no idea I had developed sensitivities to as well as foods that increased my mucous and made my symptoms worse. I had no idea I was making it worse! After treatment and detoxification, my chronic sinus infections finally cleared up and didn't return. No more antibiotics were needed and I was able to lose 20 pounds without feeling like I was on a diet. My energy even grew. I didn't realize I had low energy because of this chronic sinus condition.

Testimonial #11

I suffered seasonal spring allergies for years. I managed with over the counter medications but they made me feel sluggish, hungry and irritable. But last year it peaked and my symptoms were the most severe. A friend insisted I go to Immune Matrix for an evaluation and I found out that certain sugars made my grass allergies worse. I have to admit I do have a sweet tooth but nothing out of the ordinary so I was astounded to hear this. My allopathic allergy doctor never mentioned this. After less than 10 treatments I am allergy and medication free! It was so simple I regret not coming sooner. My head is clear, I don't crave sugars anymore and I even had enough energy to go join a gym for some classes.

Testimonial #12

My multiple chemical sensitivities were so severe my husband bought me a cabin to live in isolation. We lived separate like this for 7 years until Anna Manayan flew out to evaluate and treat me. She found my detoxification pathways were compromised by chronic toxic retention. That is what she called it. I sort of figured that was the case because I managed to detoxify only with coffee enemas and was not getting better just coping. After embarking on the slow road to reversing these immune sensitivities, I was able to go away to a bed and breakfast with my husband for the first time in 7 years. I'm astounded. My strength and vitality is getting stronger every day. I no longer live in isolation and avoidance. I've moved back into our home.

Testimonial #13

I suffered from seasonal allergies so severely that upon waking I'd sneeze uncontrollably. My eyes would water and I couldn't put my make up on. The anti-histamines made me so sleepy that taking notes in school was nearly impossible. I noticed my medications were beginning to wear off an hour earlier so I was having to take more than the recommended dose to suppress my symptoms. I was feeling very drugged and sleepy. In desperation I was willing to try anything and began treatments with Immune Matrix. I discovered I was so toxic, had sugar sensitivities and many food and hormone sensitivities. I had no idea what a mess I was. The outcome though was elimination of my seasonal allergies, unexpected elimination of the recurring eczema on my hands that I had since childhood and the delightful cure of my endometriosis that had already required two surgeries with possibly a hysterectomy in my future were it not for Immune Matrix! The biggest surprise is that with the coming of the allergy season I am allergy free and my monthly cramps and fatigue from my menstrual cycle are gone! I can run my 10K's without suffering cramps and I no longer feel exhausted, bloated or cranky before my periods.

Testimonial #14

I'm in my mid-fifties and my energy was just getting less and less. I tried being more active but that exhausted me. I tried being vegan but that drained me of my energy. I tried sleeping more and that didn't improve anything. My M.D. wanted to put me on an anti-depressant and I tried a few different ones with no change in my symptoms. After my initial evaluation with Immune Matrix, I was overwhelmed. It was now starting to make sense. I had low grade bacterial infections in my gums that I thought were just normal gum irritation. But this infection was wearing down my entire body. It had caused my digestive system to have the wrong flora, leading to the development of leaky gut that lead to food sensitivities that further made me insulin resistant and tired after eating. That in turn wore down my adrenal gland and so I became easily fatigued. It seemed like one thing after another but I embarked on their program to deal with each issue and now my brain clarity and energy is like night and day. I sleep so much better and I have the active social life I had almost given up for lack of any answers.

Testimonial #15

I had a history of asthma on and off my entire life. It came back and I was given an inhaler to control symptoms as much as I hate using it. I had to, especially before bed. After a few weeks of this I began to have problems staying asleep and would wake up I was told during the hours when the liver was most active according to Chinese Medicine. It sort of made sense. The interruptions in my sleep cycle were taking a toll on my days. I felt so sleepy during the day I'd have to nap and had trouble focusing on reading at my job. However, after my initial evaluation with Immune Matrix I knew why this was happening. The prescription medication was the straw that stressed my liver's capacity to keep up with processing toxins. I had developed more food, environmental and mold allergies than I was aware, and it was because I had become more toxic. I embarked on their detoxification and treatment program and soon I didn't need to take my inhaler, I was no longer having episodes of wheezing. The triggers were disappearing and now I no longer need my inhaler. I've been inhaler and symptom free for over five years now.

Testimonial #16

I thought I was having problems sleeping because I would wake up tired more and more. The odd thing was that a new job had me traveling and I found I slept better when away from home when most people say the opposite. A friend of mine told me to get evaluated at Immune Matrix because if anyone could figure things out they could. I was astounded, I had two issues that sound very unusual but I was advised that it does occur. It's just not widely known. I had developed an immune sensitivity to my husband's chemistry. We tested me against his hair and my immune system reacted. Sleeping next to him all night was making me feel drained by morning, while away I didn't experience this drain on my energy. I also found out that I had developed a sensitivity to EMFs, things like computers, TV, microwave frequencies all fatigued my body.

After receiving treatment, these bizarre symptoms no longer plague me. My husband doesn't understand it but is happy I feel better and wake up refreshed.

ABOUT THE AUTHOR

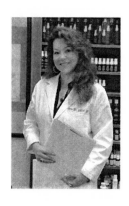

Anna Manayan, J.D., Dipl.Ac., L.Ac., NBIMA, Dipl.ABAAHP , a nationally recognized integrative/ alternative medical practitioner, featured on national TV, MSNBC & CNN, voted 'Best of the Bay' Alternative Doctor in San Francisco Bay Area and Covington's Executive of the Year 2012, has traveled extensively around the world to learn, research and seek answers for her patients. Her investigations have helped her to learn and develop innovative techniques to get to the root of immune and metabolic issues. With diligent trial and error she has brought her collective knowledge and research to her patients via her Immune Matrix clinics.

Patients come to see her from all over the globe on their own and via referral from their physicians. She will work with your doctor to help optimize your body's response to a treatment protocol and to uncover previously unseen causes. Her specialty is the treatment of the most challenging cases of chronic fatigue, multiple chemical sensitivities, bizarre unsuspected immune pathologies, Lyme disease, chronic viral and very metabolically challenged patients whose brain chemistry and digestive states are so poor that their doctors cannot give them supplements or medications without them reacting.

Anna's expertise in computerized diagnostics, detoxification, drainage & bio-energetic metabolic/immune therapy puts her in a unique position to reset the body's metabolic and immune systems to establish balanced hormonal, neurotransmitter, metabolic and immune based biochemical pathways.

In addition to overseeing multiple clinics, she travels extensively across the United States, Canada, and UK lecturing and assisting in the treatment of severely immune compromised patients too ill to travel for treatment. Her energy, dedication and passion to help people optimize their health by integrating their biochemical, energetic, structural, & emotional aspects of dis-ease is readily apparent with your first consultation.

Anna's passion in uncovering the cause for what plagues our bodies is not limited to disease and chronic illness. She is also passionate about optimizing one's health. As a diplomat with A4M (American Academy of Anti-Aging Medicine), she brings innovative medical advances to her patients daily to optimize their health. Telomere therapy to determine the rate your genes have been damaged by lifestyle and disease and reversing the damaging, gene repairing skin care products, organic baby skin creams, natural cellulite reversals and the **Immune System Weight Loss Program**, a metabolic/immune weight loss and maintenance program that *breaks through* weight loss barriers unlike anything in the country, are all a part of Immune Matrix's getting healthy and optimizing one's health missions.

Her passion and energy doesn't end there. Patient education is a pet peeve and passion and so she is an avid author of articles published regularly about the clinical findings of her research and practice. Her articles can be found on her blog www.chronicfatigueandnutrition.com.

With knowledge there is power to change! Soon she will be hosting a radio station entitled Optimum Health Radio to feature passionate and trend setting practitioners and treatment modalities in integrative, functional and alternative medicine! (www.optimumhealthradio.com)

As an attorney, she donates her time freely when needed to assist on legal matters concerning expanding insurance coverage for alternative medical care, acupuncture, scope of practice, peer review, and rules and regulations regarding the use of herbal medicine and medical devices.

Social Media:

Blog: http://www.chronicfatigueandnutrition.com
Website: http://www.yourlowenergytrap.com
Twitter: http://www.twitter.com/immunematrix
Facebook: http://www.facebook.com/annamanayan/immunematrix
Linkedin: http://www.linkedin.com/annamanayan
Radio: www.optimumhealthradio.com
Immune Matrix: 888-519-5755

RESOURCES

Anna Manayan/Immune Matrix Clinics
888-519-5755
www.chronicfatigueandnutrition.com

American Academy of Anti-Aging Medicine
www.worldhealth.net
888-997-0112

Apex Energetics
www.apxenergetics.com
800-736-4381

Diagnos-Techs™
www.diagnostechs.com

Energetix
www.goenergetix.com
Epigenic Research
www.epigenicresearch.com

Immune System Weight Loss
www.immunesystemweightloss.com
https://www.facebook.com/pages/Immune-System-Weight-loss-Program/1384532471786645

Immune Matrix
www.immunematrix.com
Metagenics
www.metagenics.com

NET
www.netmndbody.com
800-888-4638

Optimum Health Radio,
Your Trusted Source for Optimum Health
www.optimumhealthradio.com

SpiroStat
USA 806-885-2929

FURTHER READING:

Metabolic/Immune articles:

www.chronicfatigueandnutrition.com

Genotype Nutrition

Dr. D'Adamo

www.4yourtype.com

The Brain Chemistry Plan

Dr. Michael Lesser

http://www.cancercontrolsociety.com/bio2002/lesser.html

Thyroid Power

http//www.thyroidpower.com

Virtual Medicine

By Dr. Keith Scott-Mumby

www.scott-mumby.com

Why Do I Still Have Thyroid Symptoms

Dr. Datis Kharrazian

www.thyroidbook.com